Praise for
The Mud & The Lotus

"A comprehensive and unique guide to the basics of yoga for students and teachers. Highly recommended!"

—**Larry Payne**, PhD, C-IAYT, E-RYT500. Founding Director, Yoga Therapy Rx™ and Prime of Life Yoga™. Co-author, *Yoga for Dummies*, *Yoga Rx*, and *Yoga Therapy & Integrative Medicine*.

"I highly recommend *The Mud & The Lotus* to anyone currently teaching yoga, or thinking of entering this highly rewarding field. Interest in studying to become a Registered Yoga Teacher has only grown over the past several years and with it, the preponderance of books and training guides, all approaching the practice and business of becoming a teacher from different angles. One of the most challenging things for teachers, especially new teachers, is to find one guide that can lead them through their careers, taking into account all aspects of being a teacher: teaching, conducting yourself as a teacher, running a business (be it a studio or as an independent teacher), and understanding all the components of the practice itself (poses, breathing techniques, alignment, anatomy, and so on). Butler provides teachers—new and experienced— one guide that can support them throughout their careers. Her book will mentor new teachers, helping them pull together all they learned in training, adding essential pieces not presented. It will be a reminder to more senior teachers in some areas, raising new aspects of yoga for further growth. Personal stories lend an authentic and warm vibe, so it really feels like Butler is right there with you, supporting you as you develop."

—**Karen Fabian**, MS, E-RYT. Founder, Bare Bones Yoga. Author, *Stretched* and *Structure and Spirit*.

"A wonderfully practical—and inspiring—foundations book based upon Butler's years of caring experience in the real world. The title is quite appropriate, as Butler weaves in many personal highs and lows that most of us will relate to, and shares examples of how her yoga practice helps. Her chapter "Yoga Business Basics" will be especially valuable to many, with much pragmatic education not readily found elsewhere. Her "Yoga Lifestyle" chapter flows naturally and authentically from her teachings and experiences. Highly recommended for the beginning or aspiring yoga teacher. "

—**John Kepner**, MA, MBA, C-IAYT. Executive Director, International Association of Yoga Therapists (IAYT).

The Mud & The Lotus

A Guide and Workbook for Students of Yoga

COURTNEY DENISE BUTLER

et alia
press

Little Rock, Arkansas

2017

Published in the United States of America by:
Et Alia Press
1819 Shadow Lane
Little Rock, AR 72207
etaliapress.com

ISBN: 978-1-944528-92-8
Library of Congress Control Number: 2017910151

Edited by Erin Wood
Cover Image illustration by David McBurney: *Lotus from the mud*
Cover & Layout Design by Amy Ashford, Ashford Design Studio, ashford-design-studio.com
Illustrations by Elizabeth Hartzell
Photographic images of author in poses by Meredith L. Finn, SouthernRouteDesign.com
Indexing by Kathryn Oliverio

Dedicated to my yoga teachers, Robin Johnson and Elana Johnson,
with love, respect, and deep honor.

A Note on the Cover Image
from David McBurney

My mother's name means "lotus" in Vietnamese. The lotus is also the National flower of Vietnam. I love the Buddhist story—which reminds me of my Vietnamese grandmother—of how a lotus can represent life and growth from the dark muddy depths of a river, reaching up into the sunlight, and finally opening to the sky with one of the most beautiful flowers. This image is for all the mums (and mums of mums) out there.

The Mud & The Lotus

A Guide for Students of Yoga

Courtney Denise Butler

C- IAYT, 500 E-RYT, RCYT, RPYT, YACEP, POLY-500, Y12SR

Table of Contents

The Mud & The Lotus
A Guide for Students of Yoga

Preface *i*

Letter to Readers i

My Lineage iii

Section 1: Overview *1*

What is Yoga? 1

The Eight Limbs of Yoga 1

Types of Yoga 2

The Five Points of Yoga 3

A Brief and Basic History of Yoga 4

Yoga Masters of India 6

Modern Day Western Teachers 7

Section 2: The Practice of Teaching *11*

Credentialing 11

Structuring a Class: The Bell Curve Method 13

Permission Language 16

Styles of Hatha Yoga 16

Music 18

Section 3: Limbs 1 and 2, Yamas and Niyamas *21*

Ethics and Yoga 21

Understanding and Being Your Authentic Self 24

Expectations of Practice and Teaching 27

Understanding the Student...28

Section 4: Physical and Energetic Anatomy *33*

Physical Anatomy/Systems of the Human Body.................................33

Energetic Anatomy 39

Mantras, Mudras, and Bandhas 47

Gunas 49

Basics of Energetic Anatomy...49

Section 5: Limbs 3 and 4, Pranayama and Asana *51*

Pranayama..51

Asana..53

Props...55

The Poses 56

    Easy Seated Pose — Sukhasana 61

    Staff — Dandasana 62

    Cobbler — Baddha Konasana 63

    Lateral Side Leans — Ardha Parighasana 64

    Seated Spinal Twist — Paravritta Sukhasana 65

    Cat–Cow — Durga–Go 66

    Child's Pose — Balasana..67

    Down Dog — Adho Mukha Svanasana..68

    Standing Forward Fold — Uttanasana 70

    Mountain — Tadasana 71

    Warrior 1 — Vira 1 72

    Warrior 2 — Vira 2 73

Triangle — Trikonasan 74

Pyramid — Parsvottanasana 75

Wide-Legged Forward Fold — Prasarita Padottanasana..............76

Chair — Utkatasana...77

Tree — Vrkshasana...78

Locust — Shalabhasana 79

Cobra and Sphinx — Bhujangasana..80

Seated Forward Bend & Half Seated Forward Bend — Paschimottanasana ... 81

Shoulder Stand & Half Shoulder Stand — Sarvangasana and Viparita Karani..82

Bridge — Setu Bandhasana 83

Reclined Spinal Twist Series — Jathara Parivartanasana............84

Knees to Chest — Apanasana 86

Corpse — Shavasana 87

Section 6: Limbs 5 through 8, Pratyahara, Dharana, Dhyana, and Samadhi *89*

Limb 5 — Pratyahara 90

Limb 6 — Dharana 91

Limb 7 — Dhyana...92

Limb 8 — Samadhi 95

Meditation in Practice...95

Section 7: Yoga Business Basics *97*

Finding Work and Getting Paid 97

Gyms and Colleges...98

Studios..98

For Studio owners, Prospective Owners, and Teachers................99

Determining Per Class Charge 103

Income Sources for Yoga Teachers 103

Working with Other Businesses: The Percentage Approach....................105

Private Lessons, Intensives (Events), Parties, and Corporate Yoga 107

Summing up Financials and Where to Teach 109

Advertising and Marketing Ethically 109

Marketing Budgets 111

Studio Location 113

Business Ethics in the Yoga World 113

Section 8: The Yoga Lifestyle *117*

Living a Happy Life with Yoga 118

Section 9: Sample Classes and Guidelines *121*

Sample Class - Illustrated Example 122

Sample Class 2 - Photo Example 124

Biobliography *127*

The Mud & The Lotus
A Workbook for Students of Yoga

Section 1: Overview *133*

Section 2: The Practice of Teaching *139*

Section 3: Limbs 1 and 2, Yamas and Niyamas *145*

Section 4: Physical and Energetic Anatomy *149*

Section 5: Limbs 3 and 4, Pranayama and Asana *157*

Section 6: Limbs 5 through 8 *177*

Section 7: Yoga Business Basics *179*

Section 8: The Yoga Lifestyle *187*

Section 9: Sample Classes and Guidelines *193*

Workbook Key *197*

Acknowledgements *205*

About the Author *211*

Preface

Dear Friends,

Thank you for choosing *The Mud & The Lotus*.

The life cycle and symbolism of the glorious lotus flower have inspired many for centuries, myself included. Lilting gently on the surface of the water, the lotus appears pristine and fragile. However, its journey to this state of beauty begins as it sprouts from the depths of the mud below it. Out of the muck and through dingy waters, it rises toward the water's surface and the sun. It first glimpses light as a small flower pod and then, as its stem grows and strengthens, it bursts forth and opens, pure and bright, to bloom and receive the sun's warmth. The beauty we see, therefore, is only part of the story. Beneath the surface, the murky water and mud continue to hold the lotus fast, anchoring it. This anchor cannot be released, for if it is, the lotus would drift and whither. Like the lotus, we are all born of suffering, of strife, of mud. Yet if we strive toward the light of growth by opening radiantly, from the mud we will rise, receiving the warmth that surrounds us and sharing our beauty with others.

My yoga practice began decades ago, yet every day I realize how much I don't know, how much there is to learn. I realize that there is continual work to be done to rise forth from the muck and transform our experiences into learning, growth, and light. The practice of yoga would take literally lifetimes to master, and life itself is a practice.

In 2008, I opened my first yoga school. At that time, I created a workbook and manual for my students. As the years passed I edited these writings, and kept journals of what I taught or learned. Over the years, students who had previously been to yoga school would come through mine again to learn more about a subject. As I traveled, teaching and taking workshops, I also noticed many workshop participants had attended yoga schools but were not teaching or were returning for clarification on the basics of yoga. I knew there was a way to write a book that would build a good foundation for a yoga student or teacher to enhance their practice and teaching (if they choose to teach). That is my intent in writing *The Mud & The Lotus* and sharing it with you.

Often, I tell my students in our schools that my goal in the 200-hour program is much like a builder constructing a house—I can provide the foundation, walls, roof, and inner workings, but how you decorate the house is up to you, is unique, and varies widely. If a person chooses to teach after school, their teaching can take on its own personality. It has never been my goal to make little carbon copies of myself, but instead to shape competent teachers who have a working knowledge in history, philosophy, ethics, lifestyle of a yogi, asana, pranayama, meditation, and how to keep themselves and others safe in the practice.

This guide alone does not qualify one to lead others. Leaders should have experience with all limbs of yoga before embarking on teaching others. One must experience for themselves the many, varied aspects of yoga to be able to transmit their knowledge effectively, and injury can occur if prior training is not taken seriously. It is my intent that when using this book for curriculum, the total training period would last eight to nine weekends, culminating in student-teachers leading a full hour of teaching the final two weekends. Progressing through one section per weekend, I ask student-teachers to begin diagramming postures immediately, three to four postures per weekend. Aside from my own teaching through the book, I ask that they share aloud with each other, and eventually teach increasingly longer segments themselves in small groups. If possible, request that they read the first two chapters of this book prior to the beginning of training. This has been a very effective method in my school for building confidence in teaching.

The practice of all facets of yoga provides awareness that we are not our thoughts or circumstances alone, and that we can change both for our own good. (I see the truth of this in my current work as a Stress Management Specialist with the Dr. Dean Ornish Heart Disease Reversal Program, empowering others to transform their health.) The practice of yoga has taught me that pain and sadness can coexist with happiness and joy. Suffering is part of life, but yoga gives us the tools to cope with that inevitable suffering and find peace and joy by looking inward. It is comforting to know that yoga is always there for me. I don't need anything outside of myself to practice. The connection is inside me; it's inside us all. Yoga teaches us to connect to ourselves, and through ourselves to others. For me, yoga has been life's greatest gift. It has enabled me to grow and find happiness in the muddy waters of life.

Whether you are using *The Mud & The Lotus* for personal growth, to teach, or to train others, I hope you enjoy it and learn something new.

Love and Light,

Courtney Butler
C-IAYT, ERYT 500, RCYT, RPYT, YACEP, POLY–500, Y12SR
Owner/ Director Balance Yoga and Wellness
Co-Owner Balance Barre
Stress Management Specialist, Dr. Dean Ornish Reversal Program

A note on the use of "I" and "We" throughout the text. For many years, I taught yoga classes and teacher trainings and workshops alone. Then as my business as a yoga teacher and trainer of yoga teachers grew I contracted with many individual yoga teachers and other professionals in related fields to assist me with teaching. You may see the wording go from "I" to "We" during times when others have assisted me as I want to give credit to the fact that this journey is sometimes internal, but other times is a collective of individuals connected through this practice.

My Lineage

Krishnamacharya is the yoga teacher by whose lineage I am most influenced. Most of my teachers over the years have come from this lineage, though it is common for yoga teachers to study with many different gurus or teachers. Many of my teachers have also studied with or been influenced by Yogananda or other teachers.

One discovers lineage by looking at the history of one's teachers and the teachers before them, as if looking at the branches of a family tree. I've had many teachers over my lifetime and most have studied with those trained by either Krishnamacharya himself or students of his son, Desikachar. My primary teachers, Robin Johnson and Elana Johnson, studied with Erich Shiffman and Rod Stryker. Shiffman was trained by several teachers including J. Krishnamurti, and would eventually train with Desikachar and B.K.S. Iyengar, who was Krishnamacharya's student.

Rod Stryker began his studies with Kavi Yogaraj Mani Finger and his son Yogiraj Alan Finger of Ishta Yoga. Kavi Yogaraj Mani Finger was introduced to yoga by Yoganananda. However, it is said that in the senior Finger's youth at age four, he met Gandhi, and during that meeting, Gandhi professed that the Senior Finger would become a teacher and philosopher.

Krishnamacharya's first teacher was his father. At the age of 28, Krishnamacharya traveled to Tibet to study with Sjt. Rammohan Guru Maharaj. The text that was handed down to him in Tibet, the *Yoga Korunta*, is said to have been later eaten by ants. Krishnamacharya taught yoga philosophy in India and he was asked to teach yoga to the students in the school and have them perform asanas for royalty. Krishnamacharya was a wrestler and gymnast himself. As he aged and saw clients one on one, he became more focused with the practice as it met the individual. I now teach what Larry Payne, PhD, refers to as the "contemporary teachings of Krishnamacharya," or his later method of teaching. I give Larry Payne, credit for giving me the words to express the way we have been teaching since I opened my school. Our focus has always been on serving the students and their needs. If we stand strong on the tenets of yoga, especially to do no harm (Ahimsa), I believe this evolution of asana is inevitable, and that it will continue to grow and change whether or not we all agree on what that change should look like.

The Mud & The Lotus

A Guide for Students of Yoga

Section 1: Overview

What is Yoga?

Yoga is difficult to define. The word yoga means "to unite or yoke together." It can also translate to mean "discipline." The root word of yoga is "yuj," which means "to bind together." The date of origination is believed to be more than 6,000 years ago in the Indus Valley in India. An individual male practitioner of yoga is called a "yogi." An individual female should be referred to as a "yogini." Males and females together are called "yogis."

Many people are drawn to yoga for its physical benefits, such as flexibility and strength. However, others are initially drawn to yoga for its stress-relieving benefits. Yoga is now commonly recommended to people by physicians and mental health professionals.

Many who come to yoga find themselves practicing for life, as yoga is adaptable to any age or ability. Since yoga would take lifetimes to fully understand, any aspect of it can become a lifelong pursuit. It teaches us that we are not one-dimensional individuals. We have emotional, physical, spiritual, and energetic bodies. Like the four legs of a chair, when one part is out of balance, the whole person will feel off center.

The continuing practice of yoga allows us to take the practices discussed in this book and use what we understand to live lives of balance and self-care. We need not be experts; there is always more to learn, even after decades of practice. Yoga is a journey, not a destination. Enjoy the journey.

The Eight Limbs of Yoga

There are eight limbs of yoga codified in the ancient text of the *Yoga Sutras* by Patanjali, written around 200 to 300 BCE. This eight-fold path provides a structure and guidelines for living a meaningful life. Practicing them is practicing the "Royal Path" or raja yoga (see below).

1. **Yamas** — Ethical and moral conduct (I often tell my students the yamas reflect how you treat others, your behavior in society, your integrity, "you're your ethics.")
   - Ahimsa — Nonviolence
   - Satya — Truthfulness
   - Asteya — Non-stealing
   - Brahmacharya — Moderation
   - Aparigraha — Nonattachment

2. **Niyamas** — Observances and Disciplines (It may help to think of this as "Me Yamas"— the ethics of how you are internally or with yourself.)
   - Saucha — Cleanliness
   - Santosha — Contentment
   - Tapas — Discipline or practice
   - Svadhyaya — Spiritual Study
   - Ishvara Pranidhana — Surrendering to a higher power.

3. **Asana** — The postures.

4. **Pranayama** — The breathing techniques.

5. **Pratyahara** — Withdrawal of the senses; Pratyahara is often taught as focusing first on the senses and then releasing.

6. **Dharana** — The ability to focus on an object, internally or externally, otherwise known as concentration.

7. **Dhyana** — Meditation, the act of focusing for a period.

8. **Samadhi** — The state of bliss. Samadhi is often described as becoming one with all beings or union with the Divine (the God of your understanding).

Teaching Tips:
Ask students to study the Yamas and Niyamas independently, online or via other texts, and follow with a group discussion.

Invite a leader to discuss the meaning of each limb and give an example from their understanding. Or ask students to study these limbs and consider together how they might be applied to daily life.

Types of Yoga

There are many types of yoga. Yoga is often seen in the West as postures, although this is a misconception made popular by the western practice of yoga as primarily posture-focused. Yoga is the connecting or yoking of the mind and/or body with something else—primarily a supreme consciousness, the God of your understanding, or a connection to the true self. Mind-body is a common term in yoga, because although in the West we often think of the two as separate entities, yoga shows us that they work in unison. That connection may be achieved through hatha yoga or the selfless service of karma yoga. Below is a list and very basic descriptions of some of the most common types of yoga.

- **Karma** — The act of selfless service. The yoga of action.
- **Bhakti** — Devotional yoga, often including prayer, chanting, singing, and ceremonies. Bhakti is the type of yoga most often said to be practiced in India.
- **Jnana** — Study of sacred scriptures. Jnana can include philosophical readings, sacred texts, intellectual debates, and other similar study methods.
- **Tantra** — Yoga of absorption or rituals, including Kundalini Yoga.
- **Mantra** — Yoga of potent sound.
- **Raja** — Often referred to as the "Royal Path." The journey toward personal enlightenment, which includes all the yogic paths. In addition, it integrates the eight limbs. Hatha yoga is represented under raja yoga.
- **Hatha** — Developed from raja yoga, hatha means "sun" and "moon," emphasizing the balancing of opposites. Although hatha emphasizes primarily a physical practice of asana (the 3rd limb) and pranayama (the 4th limb), it is not uncommon for teachers to incorporate all 8 limbs into a class in some fashion. It is a common misconception that hatha yoga means gentle yoga, but this is not necessarily the case. Whether gentle or challenging in nature, all yoga classes that include breath work, postures, and meditation are forms of hatha yoga.

Teaching Tip:
For a deeper understanding, show the documentary *Enlighten Up* and discuss it. For some, watching a film is a more effective way to learn than merely reading or hearing about yoga.

The Five Points of Yoga

Swami Vishnudevananda (1927–1993) of Kerala, India, who established the Sivananda Yoga Teacher Training Course and whose books established him as an authority on hatha and raja yoga, condensed the essence of yoga teachings into five principles for physical and mental health as well as spiritual growth. This is often helpful to new students to introduce them to a basic understanding of a yoga lifestyle.

1. **Proper Exercise** — Asana as a vehicle for proper exercise.
2. **Proper Breathing** — Practice of pranayama.
3. **Proper Relaxation** — Shavasana, and learning to detach from material possessions and worry.
4. **Proper Diet** — A clean, healthy diet.
5. **Positive Thinking and Meditation** — Finding joy in the positive, such as books, affirmations, and exposing yourself to positive outlets. Meditation through concentration and focus.

A Brief and Basic History of Yoga

The ancient wisdom of yoga is derived from many sources, including Eastern philosophy and religion. Yoga references many texts, including ancient texts, originating in the traditions of Hinduism, Jainism, Buddhism, and other religions. Yoga is generally considered a lifestyle and not a religion, and it can be practiced in a secular or spiritual way; its practices can be used to enhance one's spiritual life regardless of religion—physically, philosophically, theoretically, spiritually, or otherwise.

Regardless of approach, yoga can be referenced for guidelines on living a balanced and contented life. As discussed earlier in this text, "yoga" comes from the root word "yuj," which means to yoke or bind together. Yoga is a mind-body practice. While we know the poses themselves can help balance the body through the system of the nadis (energy channels) and chakras (energetic wheels throughout the body), we also know that yoga is a way to bring health and vitality or balance to the body on holistic level as well. Throughout yoga's history, focuses have shifted to different aspects of this ancient practice.

There is much debate on how old yoga is, especially the originating dates of the postures, or asanas. After years of research, I don't think it is possible to pinpoint a date because questions still surround the dating of some of the ancient texts, and sages (or gurus) have been passing down wisdom orally for centuries, but it is safe to say that yoga is several thousand years old.

Many of the postures we do today are a hybrid of what is believed to have been passed down from teacher to student for thousands of years. The *Hatha Yoga Pradipika*, one of the early yoga texts, describes asana like this: "Being the first accessory of Hatha Yoga, asana is described first. It should be practiced for gaining steady posture, health, and lightness of body." The *Hatha Yoga Pradipika* presents only fifteen postures. *The Yoga Sutras* define yoga in Sutra 1:1: "Yoga is the mastery of the activities of the mind-field. Then the seer rests in its true nature." The word "sutra" comes from the Greek word "suture," which means to thread together. Many would say yoga is the threading of the mind-body or the connection of the mind and the body to the higher self or supreme consciousness.

Many postures we see today do not have much written history beyond a few hundred years. Mostly, the postures have been logged and recorded in the 20th century. Yoga has a solid foundation in the Yamas, Niyamas, and the remaining eight limbs, but the physical practice of asana continues to evolve as it grows in popularity.

The history of yoga can be divided into four time periods: the Vedic, the Pre-Classical, the Classical, and the Post-Classical. Some also add a fifth period designated "Modern Yoga" into which fall Sri Krishnamacharya (my lineage), his son Desikachar, and Krishnamacharya's brother-in-law, B.K.S. Iyengar, founder of Iyengar Yoga.

Below are abbreviated highlights from each period; the study of each could consume a lifetime. I suggest the following as jumping off points for further inquiry and study.

Vedic Period

The Vedic Period was from roughly 2000 to 1000 BCE. The Vedas are among the world's oldest sacred texts, and the oldest scriptures of Hinduism, written in Sanskrit. They are said to have been created by sages following long periods of meditation. Veda means "knowledge" in Sanskrit. The four Vedas include hymns, mantras, and other texts passed down orally.

- Rig-Veda — Praise or Knowledge
- Atharva-Veda — Rituals
- Yajur-Veda — Sacrifice
- Sama-Veda — Chants

Pre-Classical Period

This period is marked by the Upanishads, a collection of more than 200 sacred Sanskrit writings containing some of the central philosophical concepts of Hinduism. (Some of these concepts are shared with Buddhism and Jainism.) The texts were probably written between 800 and 500 BCE. In one translation, Upanishad is derived from upa (near), ni (down), and shad (to sit), reflecting students sitting down near a teacher to learn from this doctrine. The Upanishads are considered part of the wisdom of the Vedic heritage, as opposed to the ritual of the Vedic heritage. They emphasized sacrifice of the ego through self-knowledge, action (karma yoga), and wisdom (jnana yoga).

Approximately 500 BCE, the *Bhagavad Gita* (translated "Lord's Song") was composed and named. It tells the story of a warrior prince named Arjuna who confronts a moral dilemma and is led to a better understanding through the intercession of the god Krishna. It addresses three principles: karma (generous actions), bhakti (caring dedication), and jnana (knowledge).

Teaching Tip:
Ask students to read the *Bhagavad Gita* and write about how it affected them.

Classical Period

The sage Patanjali codified the more definitive and comprehensive system of yoga as the *Yoga Sutras* around 400 CE. This text defined the Classical period as the first systematic presentation of yoga. Sutra means "thread." The thread of the "lower self" is joined together with the universal "higher self" in the *Yoga Sutras*. The *Yoga Sutras* describe the eight-fold path or eight limbs of yoga, which were intended to be memorized. Patanjali believed that each of us is composed of both spirit (purusha) and matter (prakriti), and that yoga could restore the spirit to its absolute reality. Patanjali is often considered the father of yoga and his Yoga Sutras still influence most styles of modern yoga. The *Yoga Sutras* include 195 yoga aphorisms (or observations, general truths), offering guidelines for a meaningful and purposeful life.

Pantajali's aphorisms are divided into four areas:
1. Concentration
2. Practice
3. Progressing
4. Liberation

Post-Classical Period

During the 15th Century, the *Hatha Yoga Pradipika* was composed by Swami Swatmarama, and remains one of the most outstanding authorities on hatha yoga. Some of the original yoga postures are first laid out in this text, and its primary goal was illuminating the physical disciplines and practices of hatha yoga as integrated with higher spiritual goals of meditation.

Beginning in the late 19th and early 20th centuries, this is the period of hatha yoga's rise in popularity, especially in the West as yoga masters began traveling. There is an even greater focus on the physical body, and more value is placed on understanding the connection between prana and the mind (with asanas, pranayama, and other methods being used to balance and prepare yogis for meditation). T. Krishnamacharya and Swami Sivananda had great influence over the proliferation of hatha yoga in India. Sivananda penned more than 200 yoga books and established yoga centers worldwide. Three of Krishmacharya's students (B.K.S. Iyengar, T.K.V. Desikachar, and Pattabhi Jois) would continue his legacy, bringing greater attention to hatha yoga around the globe.

Yoga Masters of India

The word "guru" is a Sanskrit word for a person who has achieved an enlightened state of being. It literally means "teacher" or "remover of darkness." It is my belief, as well as the belief of other experienced teachers, that the word guru should be left to the Indian culture, as it can be insulting when it is commandeered by those not of Indian heritage. A term often heard after the words "guru" is "ji." The term "guru ji" means to give respect to the teacher. You will also hear members of Indian culture say, "Papa Ji" or "Mama Ji." "Ji" simply is a term of respect.

"Swami" is Sanskrit for master. Swami is an honorific title given to a Hindu religious teacher.

This list by no means names every guru or swami of India; there are countless others. I've included here some of the most widely known gurus and a few basic facts about each one, in alphabetical order.

Desikachar — Son of Krishnamacharya. Known for Viniyoga, a gentle type of yoga that is specific to the individual. Died in 2016 at age 78.

B.K.S. Iyengar — Trained under Krishnamachraya. Known for his many books, including *Light on Yoga*. His style is known to rely heavily on props and utilizing precise alignment. Died in 2014 at age 96.

K.Pattabhi Jois — Trained under Krishnamacharya. Known for Ashtanga Yoga. Died in 2009 at age 93.

Sri T. Krishnamacharya — Modern day father of yoga. Known for yoga therapy. Teacher of many modern day masters. Died in 1989 at age 100.

A.G. Mohan — Student and biographer of Krishnamacharya. Known as a modern day master of yoga therapy. Founder of Svastha Yoga. (In Sanskrit, svastha refers to the state of complete health and balance.) Born in 1945 and still living as of the publication of this book.

Swami Satchidananda — Founder of Integral Yoga whose motto was: "Truth is one, paths are many." He founded Yogaville, an ashram in Virginia. Died in 2002 at age 87.

Paramahansa Yogananda — The first yoga master of India to take up permanent residence in the West. Known for the book Autobiography of a Yogi. Died in 1952 at age 59.

Teaching Tip:
Teachers discuss in more detail what you know about each guru or swami listed, or discuss any other gurus and their history with your students. The movies *Enlighten Up, Ashtanga NY, AWAKE: The Life of Yogananda*, and *Breath of the Gods* are good documentaries for developing understanding of these gurus and teachers.

Modern Day Yoga Teachers

In this section, I am including yoga teachers who have extensive experience and history in the field of yoga. Many of these are popular teachers and by no means does this include all the masterful teachers of yoga in the West.

Baron Baptiste — Known for Baptiste Yoga, a type of power yoga.

Baxter Bell — M.D., workshop leader, and teacher. Leads workshops and trainings in a variety of areas. Co-author of *Yoga for Healthy Aging: A Guide to Lifelong Well-Being*.

Bereyl Bender Birch — Known for the book *Power Yoga: The Total Strength and Flexibility Workout.*

Bikram Choudhury — Known for Bikram or hot yoga. There are 26 poses in Bikram yoga.

Bernie Clark — One of the credited founders of, teacher of, and leading authority on yin yoga.

Seane Corn —Known for vinyasa yoga and her humanitarian work. Began teaching in 1994.

Lilias Folan — Known as the "First Lady of Yoga." Her popular yoga program, Lilias, *Yoga and You* aired on PBS from 1972– 1999.

Anna Forest — Founder of Forest Yoga, a very athletic form of yoga. The teacher trainings are said to be very rigorous.

John Friend — Founded Anusara Yoga, and stepped down from its leadership in 2012.

Rolf Gates — Acclaimed author of the book *Meditations from the Mat: Daily Reflections on the Path of Yoga.* Experience also includes being an Army Airborne Ranger and social worker.

John Kepner — Yoga therapist and teacher. Director of the International Association of Yoga Therapists since 2003. He has been a student of yoga since 1971 and a teacher since 1997, and studied under A.G. Mohan and Gary Kraftsow.

Gary Kraftsow — Famous Viniyoga teacher. Known for his contribution to yoga therapy.

Judith Hanson Lasiter — Yoga teacher and physical therapist who coined the term "Restorative Yoga." Restorative yoga utilizes yoga props like blocks, blankets, and bolsters, and most poses are held for between three and twenty minutes.

David Life and Sharon Gannon — Known as the founders of Jivamukti Yoga. Jivamukti means "liberation while living."

Nikki Myers — Famous for Yoga of 12-Step Recovery known as Y12SR, she leads and trains teachers to work with yoga and the 12 steps.

Larry Payne — The founding president of the International Association of Yoga Therapists. Founding director Yoga Therapy Rx™ & Prime of Life Yoga™ programs at Loyola Marymount University, and author of many books.

Shiva Rea — Known for her specific type of yoga and dance called "trance dance." She uses music and dance combined with yoga.

Erich Shiffman — Studied under the philosophical teacher Krishnamaturi, then went to school and studied with Desikachar in the Krishnamacharya – Desikachar style of teaching. Is known for his book and video *Yoga: The Spirit and Practice of Moving into Stillness.*

Rod Stryker — Founder of Para Yoga. Has taught tantra yoga and meditation for over thirty years. Author of *The Four Desires: Creating a Life of Purpose, Happiness, Prosperity, and Freedom.*

Patricia Walden — Rose to fame with the video *Yoga for Beginners* released by *Yoga Journal.* She is a renowned Iyengar teacher.

Rodney Yee — Former dancer who rose to fame in the 1990s as a yoga teacher. He now teaches worldwide, and with his wife Colleen Saidman Yee is part of the Urban Zen teacher training.

Teaching Tip:
Leaders discuss in detail teachers you would like to highlight for further study and discussion.

Note: You may choose to proceed to *The Mud & The Lotus: A Workbook for Students of Yoga*, Section 1, at the end of this book to reinforce the concepts in this chapter, or wait until you have finished the entire book.

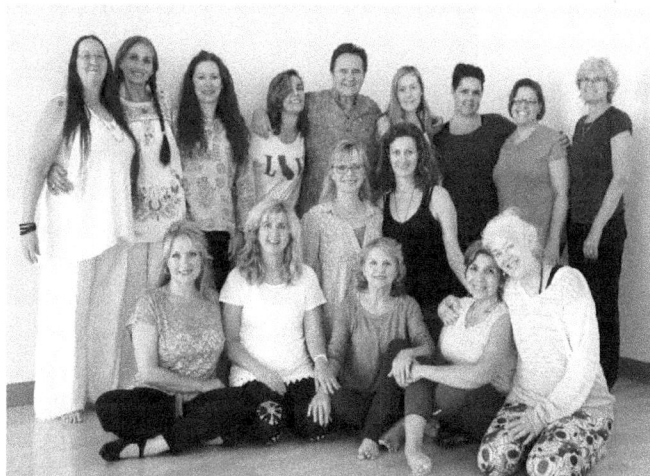

Left: The author's Prime of Life Yoga graduating class, taught by Larry Payne. To Payne's left is his sister, Lisa Galizia of Bee Cave Yoga, also a yoga teacher. Author pictured at the left front, seated.

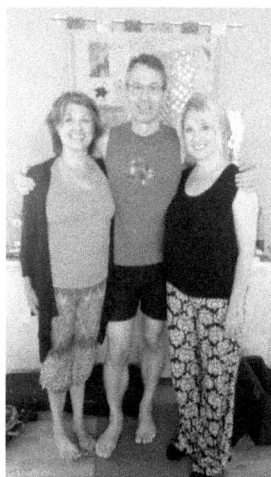

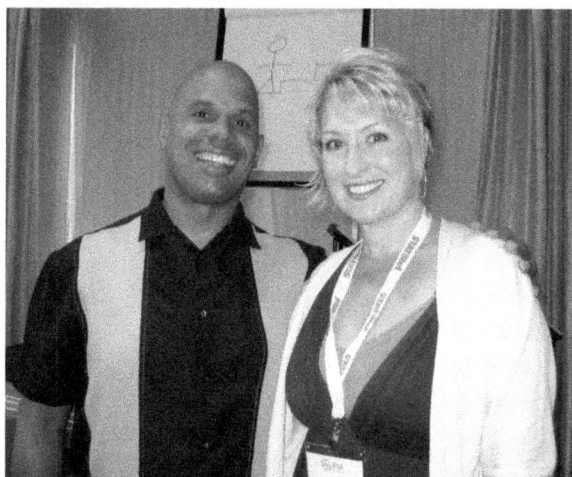

Left:
(L to R) Mary Stiles— longtime yoga teacher and friend, Dr. Baxter Bell, and Author.

Right:
Author with Rolf Gates at the Yoga Alliance Conference in Washington D.C. in 2013.

Section 2: The Practice of Teaching

Credentialing

State Licenses

As of this book's publication, some states require yoga schools to be state licensed while others do not. Schools then provide certificates to yoga teachers. Since licensing for schools changes frequently, students should check with their state Board of Career Education or the Board of Education for current information. Many of these resources can be found online, such as through the Yoga Alliance.

Yoga Alliance Credentialing

Yoga Alliance is a nonprofit organization that sets standards for yoga schools and yoga teachers, and is the largest credentialing agency of yoga teachers. Guidelines change often, so it is important to visit yogaalliance.org to see what is new. Registration as a yoga teacher or a yoga school is currently voluntary and not required to teach yoga.

Yoga Alliance has guidelines for schools to qualify for registration at several different levels. All schools issue a certificate of completion and then the student applies to Yoga Alliance for registration of their credentials should they choose to do so.

Yoga Alliance School Designations

- **RYS 200** (Registered Yoga School at the 200 hour level). The program has an accumulation of 200 hours to graduate.

- **RYS 300** (Registered Yoga School at the 300 hour level). 300-hour programs are set for students who have already attended a 200-hour program. Students who complete both a 200- and 300-hour program will qualify for an RYT 500 credential upon graduation. Students must have 100 hours of teaching before registering.

- **RYS 500** (Registered Yoga School at the 500-hour level). This program is a full 500-hour program and students will qualify for an RYT 500 credential upon graduation. Students must have 100 hours of teaching before registering.

- **RCYS** (Registered Children's Yoga School). A 95-hour curriculum that is geared toward teaching children. To register with Yoga Alliance one must first complete an RYS 200 program to be able to obtain the RCYS credential.

- **RPYS** (Registered Prenatal Yoga School). A 95-hour curriculum that is geared toward teaching pregnant and postnatal women. To register with Yoga Alliance one must first complete an RYS 200 program to be eligible to obtain the RPYS credential.

- **YACEP** – Active in 2016. Continuing Education Provider Credential. Providers must be ERYT 200 or have extensive experience in their field of study.

Yoga Alliance Teacher Designations

- **RYT 200** – Must complete an accredited RYS 200 program. Must participate in continuing education every three years to keep credentials current.

- **E-RYT 200** – An RYT 200 who has a minimum of 2 years teaching experience as well as 1000 hours teaching in the classroom.

- **RYT 500** – Must complete a 200 and a 300 training, or a 500-hour accredited program. Must teach 100 hours since completing the program to apply for an RYT 500 credential.

- **E-RYT 500** – Must be credentialed at the 500 level, taught for a minimum of 4 years, and have a minimum of 2,000 hours after receiving a 200 or 500-hour designation. 500 of those hours must be after receiving a 500 hour designation.

- **RCYT** – Must be an RYT 200 in addition to completing an accredited RYCS program.

- **RPYT** – Must be an RYT 200 in addition to completing an accredited RPYS program.

Teaching Tip:
The details of Yoga Alliance Standards can quickly become overwhelming. I generally suggest my students do this order: RYT 200, E-RYT 200 (in order to get experience and learn more about yourself as a teacher), and then any other designations such as RCYT, RPYT, or advanced 300-hour training. Eager students, enjoy the journey. No school can replace real world experience.

International Association of Yoga Therapists (IAYT)

IAYT is a professional organization committed to advancing yoga therapy education, training, and research, and the professional development of its members. IAYT's mission is to establish yoga as a recognized and respected therapy. It is currently accrediting schools in the field of yoga therapy. When one has completed IAYT- accredited yoga therapy training, they can apply to become a Certified Yoga Therapist or C-IAYT.

Structuring a Class: The Bell Curve Method

My approach to structuring a class is specific to my training and many years of teaching. This may not be the same as some other schools of thought, as each lineage has its own unique characteristics. The method I share is what has worked best for me over the years, with thousands of students in my classrooms and many I have trained to be teachers. There are many resources for teachers on my website at Balanceyogaandwellness.com and through my YouTube account by searching "Courtney Butler Yoga."

The easiest form I have found to teach a class is the Bell Curve Method, sometimes referred to as The Sandwich Method. To put it simply, all classes have three parts: a beginning, a middle, and an end. These three parts should be distinct.

All balanced yoga classes move the spine in all six directions. The six directions of the spine are:
1. Forward Bending
2. Backward Bending (backbends)
3. Lateral Bending to the Left
4. Lateral Bending to the Right
5. Twisting the Spine to the Left
6. Twisting the Spine to the Right

Always balance every pose to keep the body and mind balanced, both physically and energetically. Backbends are balanced by forward bends and twists. Forward bends are balanced by backbends and twists. Below is a narrative and guide, based on the Bell Curve Method.

> *Caution:*
> Students who have medical conditions (such as glaucoma, high blood pressure, retinopathy, or dizziness) as well as pregnant students should not do poses in which the head is below the heart (inversions). Pregnant students additionally need to avoid deep twists and deep backbends, and should never do deep inversions like headstand or shoulderstand.

Class Beginning

Always ask new students to sign a waiver before class begins. At the start of class, introduce yourself to the students and tell them what props they will need. Ask about any medical conditions. Share basic housekeeping guidelines with them, such as where to place their belongings, the location of the bathroom, etc. Make them feel at home.

Share an opening, such as asking them to set an intention for the class. One might begin with seated meditation or pranayama. After a short time with this, maybe five to ten minutes, move on to joint-opening poses that warm the body and loosen the joints. See examples below, as well as additional class samples in the charts at the back of the book.

Sample Seated Meditation/Pranayama

"Let's begin by sitting in a comfortable seated position (like Sukhasana, or easy pose). Take a seat, bring your hands to your heart, and let's take a few full rounds of breath. Inhale your hands over your head and exhale your hands back to your heart." Repeat 3 times.

"If you like, you may set your intention for this class. Think about what you need in your life, what your focus is, or what words may be speaking to you today. You may dedicate your practice to someone, your own self-care, or simply set an intention to be present for this hour of practice."

Sample Joint-Opening Poses

"Next, let's proceed with some postures to warm your body."

Postures here would start either with the head or the feet. Neck loosening postures could include taking the ear to the shoulder, then taking the head to the front and back. Move on to some shoulder shrugs. Move the elbows and wrists. From here, work the waist in a lateral side lean, then a simple seated twist. Take the legs out in front into a simple cobbler pose. From here do a seated cat and cow. Lastly, flex and point the feet and move the ankles.

"From here, bring yourself to all fours in a tabletop position and let's move the body in circles at the hips and shoulders. Now inhale and bring yourself into cow's tail, exhale into cat's tail. From here, stretch the right leg out into sunbird stretch and the left arm out in front. Repeat other side. Now bring your bottom back into child's pose. From child's pose come to all fours and lift your knees and hips back into downward-facing dog or an upside down V."

Class Middle

For the middle portion of class, move into standing poses, sun salutations, balance, and stronger poses. This is where the "style" of a class will likely stand apart.

If you are teaching a gentle class there may not be a lot of standing poses or they may be gentler, like half sun salutes or standing tadasana, side leans, and forward folds. For a strong class you will have more standing postures and poses like plank and side plank. For a faster moving vinyasa class, you would move with the breath to add things like standing lunges, and sun salutations.

It is important to link postures in a commonsense fashion, reducing up and down from the back to the belly or from sitting to standing. This linking is one reason I often will do prone (on the belly) positions during the flow of sun salutations. When you get to cobra or zen asana (knees, chest, chin), this is a good time to do poses like bow, sphinx, locust, and other prone postures. You can then take students back to child's pose to counter, return to down dog, and you're on your way back to standing or moving at this point without chopping up the class.

Class End

Once you have completed your middle section, which for an hour long class should last about 20 minutes, you want to bring students back to the floor in a reasonable way. This could include moving through standing>down dog> knees, or from forward fold> all fours.

Begin cooling down by adding seated poses. Try boat>half-seated forward fold>forward fold, and then transition students to their backs for an inversion like shoulderstand or plow, if those are available to your class. After this, students should come to their backs for poses like bridge, reclined cobbler, or twists and poses where legs are inverted. The class generally ends well by doing a gentle bridge supported with a block if you choose, then knees to chest and a reclined twist of some sort. Bring the knees to the chest and then gently take the legs to shavasana.

Always take your time for shavasnana. It is best to give 10 minutes or more to this part of practice. Shavasana can be lead with a variety of meditation techniques. (Please see section on meditation). Then bring the student to the right side (unless pregnant) in seed position for a few transitional breaths. Asking them to use their hands for support, transition the students up to seated with eyes closed. Some teachers will add meditation here after a silent shavasana. Feel free to be creative and develop your own style. Some teachers like to incorporate "om" and "shanti" into the final part of practice (others may open with these as well for balance). Om is the sacred sound and symbol of the universe. All things in life are said to have the same reverberation of the sacred sound "Om." Shanti means peace, and is usually said or sung three times "Shanti, shanti, shanti."

Add a few full rounds of diaphragmatic breathing and end with Namaste. There are varying translations of Namaste, but it is a signal of mutual respect to seal the practice, basically meaning *"The light (divine) in me recognizes the light in you."*

Please reference Section 9 for a deeper understanding.

Teaching Tip:
We use the right side because it is said to give a rest to the heart with less pressure on the heart. It is also representative of facing the East or the side of the rising sun. It allows the Ida nadi (yin side, considered one of the main energy channels in the body) to remain open. This allows the left nostril to remain open and is considered to be more calming to the body. However, a pregnant student needs to have more blood volume going to the heart and the left side allows for the maximum blood flow to the main artery of the heart and to the baby.

Permission Language

Permission language is given throughout class from the time the students walk in the door until the time they leave. Permission language isn't just words; it is also an attitude. It is how you make people feel. When you tell a student to listen to their body or you offer a modification, you are using permission language.

For example, if you are teaching alternate nostril breathing, and you have an asthmatic student who is uncomfortable with this, you could tell the student to simply sit and do basic belly or ujjayi breathing. Make the student feel as comfortable as possible. You might offer some suggestions like, *"Try to focus on the breath traveling up one side of your body and down the other to help with the left-right brain connection, then reverse your mental picture as you breathe."* This makes the student an active part of the process.

In asana, an example of permission language would be having a student who is large breasted and/or is curvy open their legs in forward folds to make space. In pigeon pose, the student might have the knee between the breasts to make space. Permission language makes the student feel comfortable and gives options to make yoga accessible to all. One of the most powerful things you can say is "Listen to your body."

Teaching Tip:
Explain in detail using permission language. Use terms like *"If this is available to you"* or *"If you feel like taking a different version of the posture today"* or *"Listen to what your body needs today, and realize that is different from day to day."* Explain how to give options for poses in a 1, 2, 3 fashion, or demonstrate moving from the easier version to the more challenging version. Always show the modification if students are new before embarking on the more challenging level of a certain pose. *Example 1*: Plank. I would show a knee down version then a knees up version. This would be a 1, 2 version. *Example 2*: Tree. I would show the kickstand method of the sole of the foot to ankle (arch over ankle so as not to push the joint), then the foot to inner calf, then to the inner thigh. This is a 1, 2, 3 method.

Styles of Hatha Yoga

There is a difference between "styles" of yoga and "types" of yoga. Remember that a type of yoga is the connection of self with something else. It can be connection through works, study, or practice of asana and meditation. In this book, we are referring to the type of yoga called Hatha yoga which includes the practice of breath, asana, and meditation. Yogic philosophy may be interwoven into a hatha yoga class, but it is still a hatha yoga class if it has a focus on breathing, posture, and meditation.

There are many styles of yoga within Hatha yoga. Some styles are trademarked and must not be taught unless the teacher is certified by the school that owns the trademark. To do so would be unethical (and probably illegal). If you teach in a way that pays homage to a certain style but you are not certified in that style, then you need to say you are teaching a class "inspired by" that type. It's very important to be distinct because it is technically stealing intellectual property if one calls their own class by a trademarked name. For instance, I may say I am teaching an Iyengar-inspired class, but I would not say I am teaching an "Iyengar class" because I have not been trained by Mr. Iyengar's school. In another example, I can lead a *Prime of Life®* yoga class because I am a certified and registered Prime of Life Yoga® teacher.

- **Anusara** — A certain style focusing on certain alignment principals. Anusara is trademarked.

- **Ashtanga** — Series of 6 postures. Teacher led, students must have permission to move on to next series. Ashtanga is trademarked.

- **Bikram** — Hot yoga with certain postures done in a certain order. Bikram is trademarked.

- **Children's Yoga** — Alignment is not of the most importance. Fun, learning and self-awareness are usually more of a focus. Class length is dependent on age. Not trademarked.

- **Gentle Yoga** — More postures on the ground, slower, focuses on gentle postures and may use more props. Gentle yoga is not trademarked.

- **Hot Yoga** — Yoga practiced in a heated room. Can be slow- or fast-paced. Precautions must be taken to make sure students are safe. Avoid for high blood pressure, heart issues, serious autoimmune conditions, and pregnancy due to complications that may arise from overheating. Students need to stay well-hydrated and be mindful that they will have more flexibility due to the heat. Generally, one should be mindful not to do deep inversions in a heated room. This type of yoga has more injuries and the teachers should understand what the risks are before embarking on these types of classes. Not trademarked.

- **Iyengar** — Uses many props and focuses on alignment. Iyengar is trademarked.

- **Power Yoga** — Strong yoga, often utilizing vinyasa flow, and has a more aerobic quality. Power yoga is not trademarked and is free to use.

- **Prenatal Yoga** — Ideally, a teacher should have some special training to teach prenatal yoga, which includes poses to help reduce stress on mother and child. Because of potential harm and injury, special care should always be taken. Often, these include poses that prepare the mother for childbirth. Avoid poses on the belly, deep twists, deep back bends, being on the back for extended periods of time, and inversions. The mother will go to her left side in prenatal yoga in rescue or seed position to allow for maximum blood flow. Avoid postures that restrict blood flow to the baby. Prenatal Yoga is not trademarked.

- **Prime of Life Yoga** — Yoga for those who are entering their prime or later years. Postures are modified to fit the needs of this population. This is trademarked and one must be certified to teach a Prime of Life Yoga class.

- **Restorative Yoga** — Uses many props and the postures are held. Restorative yoga is not trademarked.

- **Yin Yoga** — Student starts with cold muscles. Focus is on the joints and deep connective tissue. Postures are held for some time. Though a distinct style, yin yoga is not trademarked.

- **Y12SR** — Yoga for 12-step recovery. Somatic and cognitive approach that has been shown to be very successful in assisting with recovery from addiction, or for those who deal with addiction in their life—whether the practitioner is him/herself an addict or close to others with addictions. This is a trademarked school and should only be taught by a certified professional.

Teaching Tip:
It is a good idea to be thoughtful and specific when naming a class. Hatha yoga is not a style; rather, it is a type of yoga. Naming a class "Hatha Yoga" is not descriptive enough. Hatha can be gentle or fast, easy or challenging. Our culture has been using the term hatha to mean gentle and vinyasa to mean fast or more powerful. These are misleading terms. Vinyasa yoga is a style of hatha yoga. Vinyasa simply means moving from one posture to the next with the breath cycle or linking the breath. The true breakdown of the word Vinyasa simply means "to place in a certain way." Vinyasa can be fast or slow. A gentle class might be described as "Gentle Hatha Yoga." A gentle class might also be described as "Slow Vinyasa." I often named a class "Stress Buster"; it is a slow and gentle hatha yoga class that combines movement with breath and holding poses for a number of breaths in a gentle fashion. Creative and descriptive names often help tell the student what to expect. Be as clear as possible about the level of challenge the student can expect.

Music

There are many opinions regarding the use of music in yoga classes. Music playlists have become popular, and live music is very popular in some yoga circles now. Most of the time, seasoned teachers will choose to not use music, or to only use music at the beginning and end of class for meditation. Music, of course, is personal. Be very aware of how your music selection may meet the class.

It is always safer to choose music without lyrics. After decades of teaching, my personal preference is to use music with no words or words in Sanskrit (because likely the student does not know what they mean so they don't distract). If you are teaching, consider your students' desires and needs ahead of your own desires. If I am teaching at the heart clinic, I use very gentle music with no Sanskrit to not put off anyone who may be unfamiliar with Sanskrit or Yoga. If you choose to integrate music into your class, here are some things to consider:

1. Music's beats per minute should match the speed of the class. Shavasana is not very relaxing with a fast beat.

2. Lyrics can be uplifting and/or distracting. People will often focus on the words rather than what's happening in their bodies or minds. Words can also lift and inspire. So consider your music carefully.

3. Music should meet the mood. I have created playlists and used certain styles of music to set the mood for the class. It can be useful to have music for a theme. For instance, it might be nice to use an upbeat rock playlist for a vinyasa flow class that is in the morning or evening, or perhaps a gentle Indian flute playlist for a more relaxed and gentle class.

4. Age may be a factor in your music selection. A seventy-year-old and a twenty-year-old may have different ideas about what is good music. Find music that fits the people you are teaching.

5. You may need a license to play music. If you are charging for classes, often you will need to pay a small licensing fee to use music. That goes for Pandora as well.

Personal Story:
Music Can Distract and Detract. On two occasions recently in yoga class, music with lyrics was played. It didn't sit well with me because the song had some very tense meaning for me. It could have totally wrecked my mental state during practice, but because I have been practicing for years I was able to refocus my thoughts. Still, I would have preferred not to hear it.

Section 3: Limbs 1 and 2, Yamas and Niyamas

Ethics and Yoga

Ethics in yoga are specifically laid out in limbs 1 and 2, the yamas and niyamas, described below.

1. **Yamas** — Ethical and moral conduct (I often tell my students this includes how you treat others, your behavior in society, and your integrity.)
   - Ahimsa — Non-violence
   - Satya — Truthfulness
   - Asteya — No Stealing
   - Brahmacharya — Moderation
   - Aparigraha — Non-attachment

2. **Niyamas** — Observances and Disciplines (It may help to think of these as "Me Yamas" the ethics of how you are internally or with yourself.)
   - Saucha — Cleanliness
   - Santosha — Contentment
   - Tapas — Discipline or practice
   - Svadhyaya — Spiritual study
   - Ishvara Pranidhana — Surrendering to a Higher Power

Yoga is a lifestyle; it is not only a physical practice as many people believe today. Yoga is a path (or a set of tools) to a more content and peaceful life. Sages (teachers, gurus) passed down, orally and in written texts, practices that would enhance one's wellbeing. The truth is yoga history is a weaving of many different texts and paths. Yoga has stood many years of time-tested techniques, especially the yamas and the niyamas. Isn't it interesting how very similar ethical guidelines are found throughout history, philosophy, and many religions throughout the world? Though yoga is not a religion, many of the people who wrote the ancient texts listed in the previous chapters were from the East and came from either Hindu, Jain, or Buddhist backgrounds. The texts themselves are not a path to a religious practice, however the practices can enhance one's spiritual path regardless of one's religious background or affiliation.

The ethical practices in yoga are great guidelines for conducting yourself in all areas of your life from personal self-care and relationships to business ethics. We don't have to reinvent the wheel; we can have faith that for many thousands of years this philosophy has assisted people in leading more content and peaceful lives. If this philosophy did not work, it would have been thrown to the wayside long ago. Let's explore the ethical guidelines now in more detail.

Use the inquiries below to spark discussions on the yamas and niyamas.

Yamas — Ethical and Moral Conduct. These guidelines are intended to help students become more aware, think about how they act externally, and consider how those actions or messages affect them internally.

- **Ahimsa — Non-violence** — In your life, do you gossip? Do you live by the Golden Rule? Do you treat others as you would have them treat you? Do you take care of yourself? Are you saying negative things to yourself or about yourself?

- **Satya — Truthfulness** — Are you using your words to tell the truth? This doesn't mean being unkind, but it does mean having integrity. Do you live by a strict code of integrity even when it may mean you do not get what you want in the short term?

- **Asteya — No Stealing** — Do you give credit to other people for their own ideas? Do you try to dominate the conversation? Are you fair? Are you out for yourself or do you practice empathy?

- **Brahmacharya — Moderation** — Do you overindulge and have regrets? This can include anything from mismanagement of money to abuse of food, drugs, alcohol, or sex, not managing your time, or anything that makes you feel you are not managing your life well. If you are a person who has a lot of regrets because of impulsive actions, then practicing moderation may help. How can you practice moderation in your life? What would this look like?

- **Aparigraha — Non-attachment** — Some attachments are necessary of course, as we are attached to our family members and those we love. We need certain things in our life like food, clothing, and shelter. However, do we place an emphasis on having certain things a certain way or do we know we are important and worthy without "things?" Do we understand that though there may be discomfort and in some cases extreme pain, that we can go on in spite of loss? This is a hard concept because it can be so painful in its deepest form. Many people have made great contributions in this world out of their deepest loss. When conducting one's life, these are great questions to ask oneself: Am I doing this because of my fear of unworthiness? Do I feel I need to be a certain type of person to receive love? Am I open to new experiences? If I didn't have this or that (clothes, car, significant other, status, etc.), would I feel whole?

Niyamas — Observances and Disciplines

- **Saucha — Cleanliness.** Do you take care of yourself? Do you feel worthy of self-care? Do you respect your surroundings and keep your life free of clutter and mess? Do you respect yourself and your family enough to care for what you have? Do you practice gratitude and gratefulness for all you have been given by caring for what you have? Do you care for your body?

- **Santosha — Contentment.** Are you content in your life? Do you practice gratitude for what you have been given? When doing work of any kind, do you practice being grateful? This is often where perspective comes in. If you dislike your job, is there a way you can change your perspective while you are in it? It doesn't mean you don't look for another job; it means you focus on the positives (money for food and shelter, friendships with colleagues, etc.) rather than the negatives. This practice alone is life changing. Once you learn how to practice this in your daily life, it's amazing how the world flows to you.

- **Tapas — Discipline or Practice.** Do you find balance in your life? Are you caring for yourself in all areas of your life spiritually, in your work life, family life, and with respect to self-care? How do you do this? What can you do to start being more disciplined? Are you being realistic about the time you have? Does it help to realize that life is not "all or nothing"? Ten minutes of exercise 6 days per week is better than no exercise at all. Twenty minutes of reading to your kid 4 times per week is better than not spending quality time with your child at all and just going through the motions. We must create balance by taking time for family and friends and not being workaholics. It is often the simple daily things done with love and attention that make a difference in the quality of our lives.

- **Svadhyaya — Spiritual Study.** We are all spiritual beings. There are many religions in this world, but some people have no religious affiliation. That doesn't mean those who don't are unable to have a spiritual practice. Practice and spirituality can be in the form of self-study of philosophy, religious texts, and spiritual texts, but it does not have to be limited to these. It is important to our overall sense of health and happiness to know that we are all connected, we all feel, we have needs and wants and basic human desires. Sadness and happiness are seen in people and animals, and emotions are universal. Practice connection to nature and to other humans. Practice connection to the God of your understanding and knowing. If we feel alone in this world, we are in a sad state of affairs. If we feel a spiritual connection, we feel more interested in life. Be mindful not to isolate yourself. No one can tell you how to do this, it is uniquely in you. You may become more connected may be through church, or nature, study of spiritual texts, asana, pranayama and meditation, or other practices.

- **Ishvara Pranidhana — Surrendering to a Higher Power.** Surrendering does not mean putting your head down and giving up; it involves opening your arms and heart, and accepting that you are not fully in control. Surrendering is the basis of the Serenity Prayer, of knowing what is within your control and what is not. People come into and out of our lives, tragedies happen, people die, and things don't always make sense. At the end of the day, the only thing within our control is how we choose to live—how we manage ourselves. Accepting that we can only control ourselves is a way of surrendering. Allowing ourselves to realize what is in our control and what is not helps us to surrender. How do you practice surrendering? In your life, are there times you have had to let go and trust the universe or the God of your understanding? How did that turn out?

Saucha — Cleanliness. At a young age, my family taught me that no matter how little money we had in the bank, we could keep ourselves and our property (cars, home, land) clean and well kept. This wisdom gave us a sense of self-respect and dignity even when we were struggling financially.

Tapas — Discipline or Practice. I once heard, *"The hardest thing is getting started."* Writing this book has been challenging because I have many roles in my life. I find myself stopping and starting often to balance my life because I am a mother of four as well as a business owner, contractor, and partner. It can be difficult to find the time to write, but I make the time because I am aware that sharing this book may be helpful to someone else and it is something I feel called to do. Also, I don't want to miss out on the experience of it. Years ago I would have put myself last, postponed my projects so I could care for everyone else. This would leave me exhausted, depressed, and anxious. I realized that changing this practice in my life was like putting my oxygen mask on in a plane before putting on my child's. We must care for ourselves and our own lives before we can fully care for anyone else.

Ishvara Pranidhana — Surrendering to a Higher Power

The Serenity Prayer
God grant me the serenity
to accept the things I cannot change;
courage to change the things I can;
and wisdom to know the difference.

Recently, I heard what my friend calls *"a walk-in,"* the equivalent of experiencing a messenger from God or the universe. During a challenging moment in my life, I was floating the Caddo River when I overheard a nearby young man say to another young man, *"When bad things happen, I don't get upset anymore; I just roll with it."* I realized this is the essence of surrendering—understanding that when things happen, we don't have all the answers, but we will do the best we have with the resources we have been given and trust that there is meaning beyond our understanding.

Understanding and Being Your Authentic Self

If you do the work, yoga will open a whole new world to you beyond physical practice. Yoga offers a lifestyle, every aspect of which presents opportunities for growth, joy, and fulfillment. Trusting the methods and the practice is essential in finding the balance and peace that yoga can bring.

Slow Down and Listen

I once heard a wise man say that he was enlightened only for a few hours a day. This is a common characteristic of many who have been on this path for some time. In the movie *Enlighten Up*, the young journalist asks the wise yoga teacher (and I will paraphrase), *"Do you manage to keep your small self (wants) under control and live only in your big self (higher levels of wisdom)?"* The wise yoga master says, *"Ask my wife!"*

Years ago, I became very disheartened and confused about yoga and my place in the yoga world. I was seeing people I had once admired in positions of power being caught doing unethical things. In my own smaller yoga community, I felt disenchanted with the studio and health club where I worked. The studio was asking me to substitute teach up to ten classes a week on a regular basis, and I didn't know how to say *"No."* The health club where I had been working for many years was sold to someone who had very different vision than I was accustomed to working under. I was also working at a local college where I had four two-hour classes per week. My classes were very full, which was a good problem, but I was having a hard time keeping up with so many students. On average, I was teaching seventeen classes a week. I was drained and disheartened. This didn't seem to be what I signed up for. My personal practice was suffering and the yoga I once loved seemed far away.

I had a five-month break at the college for summer vacation, and I quit all my other teaching jobs. I was in desperate need of a break and I wasn't sure what to do, so I took some time off from *all* teaching. For five months, yoga for me was found in walks at the lake meditating on nature. I did very little asana practice at that time. I just walked and walked and swam and played with my kids and animals. I had to reconnect to life outside the yoga world. Simply put, my yoga—my mind-body connection—was found outside of asana for this time.

One day when I was walking, I came to a stop sign and I heard what I call the *"God Voice."* I describe the God Voice as something more than a random thought. The thought is so loud in your head that it takes over you, and suddenly you hear in your heart what God, the Universe, is trying to tell you. At the time it happened, I had been doing yoga for seventeen years and teaching for seven. In the months before I quit teaching I had done a series of workshops on special needs, like yoga for scoliosis. So, the voice comes over me and says, *"Teach the teachers."* I knew at that moment I was meant to open a yoga teacher training program.

My teacher Robin Johnson, who lived an hour away, was not actively running her school; she was only mentoring a few people a year. I decided before I approached her, I would see if I was capable of writing a curriculum. For nine months, I sat in my car writing curriculum while my kids went to guitar practice. When I completed the curriculum, I submitted it to Yoga Alliance to see if it would be approved. I then spent another seven months going back and forth with the review board until I was finally approved. But, and there is a big *"but,"* I would not pay my dues to Yoga Alliance nor open a school without my teacher's blessing. I called Robin and told her what had been going on. She gave me her full support and asked me to be affiliated with her school. She wrote a glowing recommendation and I was immediately granted accreditation.

During that phone call, I told Robin how disheartened I had become with the yoga community. She said, *"Courtney, anytime you put a person or a group on a pedestal, you are sure to be disappointed."* With that I realized I had put a lot of pressure on human beings to be perfect just because they practiced yoga. The lesson was, and remains today, that being imperfect is part of being human—and that goes for those who practice and teach yoga as well. We are all imperfectly perfect human beings full of flaws, and most of us are doing the best that we can. That is why it is called a yoga "practice," because we continue to practice our entire lives. What yoga gives us changes and adapts to what our needs are. Dealing with our own and others' imperfections gracefully and with patience and understanding *is* part of the yogic path.

My teachers Robin Johnson and Elana Johnson (same last names, not related) are shining examples to me of what a yogi should be. They have integrity, they live by the tenets of the yamas and niyamas. They have faith beyond measure and have always led me in the way of high moral character. They expected a lot from us as yoga teachers and we didn't want to disappoint them. To this day, the group of women I trained with have all shown a high level of moral character and ethics, and I have the utmost respect for them. As far as expectations go, I expected everyone in the yoga world to have the same moral character of my teachers whom I admired so much. But I've realized that not everyone is on the same path—we all have lessons to learn and some people will make choices that we might not understand. I try to remember not to take it personally, just to spend my energy on what I need to focus on for my own wellbeing and happiness.

My advice based on these experiences is that when one is unsure, confused, or overwhelmed, it is a good idea to slow down and listen for guidance. Once guidance is received and/or the path becomes clear, we should proceed holding ourselves to high standards, but avoid putting others on pedestals.

Contentment as a Practice
I can attest that a life lived by the values and tenets of yoga can bring fulfillment to every day. It used to be that I thought I was lucky if I felt content, meaning happiness was something I likened to dessert, like a special treat that only happened occasionally. With much sincerity, I can tell you that I now find happiness in every day. There are times when I am sad, angry, defeated, and exhausted; however, each day I experience mo-

ments of pure happiness. Why? What has changed? The change happened over time as I learned to shift my thoughts. I can go from being upset about something to stopping and being grateful for the sun hitting my shoulders or for the breeze in the air. If I allow myself to be fully present in the moment, I can detach from sadness and experience joy. Yoga has taught me this through consistent practice in the good times and the hard times.

The true test of this came to me about three and a half years ago. I was in a very challenging relationship. The end was long coming and I had done all I felt that I could do. I was out of answers. Then one day I found the strength to move forward. During that dark time, I found that through the practice of yoga I could momentarily detach from the pain. I could compartmentalize my personal life from my work life. From day one I worked and didn't have to miss because I had the tools that yoga had given me to have the strength to move forward. I kept teaching and trying to give back; this was yoga's gift to me. Through the practice of the 8 limbs of yoga, I found some happiness in every day.

That first year on my own, we were statistically in poverty, but somehow, we made it one day at a time. I learned to self care and my children, who've had some struggles, have turned out to be very smart, self-sufficient young adults. My practice helped me appreciate the moments that were good, to have compassion for myself, to learn to love myself, and to understand my own needs and my children's needs. This is the gift of appreciation and adaptation, a gift that money cannot buy. No matter what circumstances life brings, is comforting to know that yoga is always there for me, and the lessons I can learn from it are infinite.

Expectations of Practice and Teaching

I have seen so many yoga teachers struggle because they have expectations of what teaching yoga will look like, and the reality does not match those expectations. Because we practice and/or teach yoga does not mean our daily lives will be free of stress or that teaching does not come with challenges. In my experience, those who choose to teach will be best served if they think of it as a job of service rather than one for recognition of physical ability.

Teaching is great work. However, we all fall short at times and some days can be challenging when there is a difficult student or class attendance is not what you think it should be. The need for security, acceptance and validation is natural, but to retain lasting happiness we must look within and not at that person who complained because we didn't live up to their expectations or at the fact that only two students came to class. We all want to be validated in life; this is a normal human trait. It is important though to set out to share this knowledge and experience to assist others in having happy and healthy lives.

The teachers I see who are truly happy are the ones who are day in and day out serving others and who also consistently carve out time for their own practice. Those teachers feel blessed by their work, and they are usually the most successful. To paraphrase Swami Satchidananda (1914–2002), founder of *Integral Yoga*, whose life's work was dedicated to sharing the message of service to others: *when we quit worrying about who is going to take care of us and focus on service or what others need, those people then in turn care for us.* So simple, and so true.

I rest in the peace knowing that I don't need to reinvent the wheel or come up with my own profound conclusions to share with every class, rather I can be a conduit for the wealth of knowledge that has been developing for centuries. Wise people who came before gave gifts in perpetuity through the wisdom of the yamas and niyamas, as well as the other six limbs of yoga, to assist us all on this journey. Our role is listen and do the work, even when (especially when!) it is challenging. The most important work of our lives if often done in the face of adversity, and that certainly includes our teaching journey.

Teaching Tips:
As you teach, continue to ask yourself: *What is this decision based on? Am I teaching for the class that shows up, or teaching to demonstrate my own physical ability or perceived knowledge?* (One example would be teaching headstands in a room full of beginners, which clearly would not be in the best interest of a new student, in order to show off one's own headstand.) See the correlating section in the workbook for questions that will help you understand yourself better, on page 145.

Understanding the Student

In understanding your students, it is helpful to reflect on what brought you to teacher training.

Personal Stories:
My Yoga Teaching Journey
My yoga teaching journey began in the late 1990s when I was in college, finishing my degree in early childhood education. My classmates were much younger because I had been in college for nearly ten years while I was parenting three boys. At that point, my yoga practice had been a consistent part of my life for more than a decade. The women in the lab school I attended were often younger or struggling financially. One student suffered from debilitating anxiety. I could relate to her as anxiety has also been my life-long struggle. I asked her if she was interested, and simply started showing her how to do some basic breath work and yoga postures.

Some school administrators took notice of what I was doing and asked me if I would want to teach a community class. So I started my career by helping other people with what had helped me. At this time I also signed up to take a class with Elana Johnson ERYT 500 who was teaching at the college. I was already teaching yoga and doing quite well with high attendance rates in my classes at a local college and a health club. I was enjoying helping others and learning from Elana. Within a few short years I would join Robin Johnson's school, Turquoise Tree, in Benton, Arkansas. Elana and Robin had worked together and had gone to school together to achieve their credentials. I would teach for three years before graduating with my RYT 200 in 2004.

My physical ability was at its prime in my early thirties. My mom says I was born with my toes in my mouth, indicating that I was always flexible. I could practice advanced postures such as Full Pigeon and Bird of Paradise with ease. Looking back now I can see that I let my own ego get in the way sometimes, though I was unaware. Another issue was my lack of understanding of older and less flexible populations. A newspaper photographer came into class one day to get a picture of me teaching, I believe I was 32 at the time. She asked me to strike a pose while teaching, so I went into full pigeon, a very challenging pose for many people. My students laughed because they were thinking "Are you serious, lady? You expect us to do that?!" That was a humbling moment for me. I was embarrassed, my awareness suddenly in full view. That moment changed me and I became very aware that I was letting my practice be about me. People might think, "Wow look at her, I could never do that!" which could have a negative outcome. Instead, I could have done something beautiful and simple and they might think, "Wow, I think I could do that!" which could have a very positive outcome. Since that humbling day I now only allow pictures of myself in fairly accessible poses for the general population. Through Robin and Elana's teaching I began to understand the importance of having my own practice and the difference of teaching people what *they* needed not what *I* wanted to practice.

More time passed, and I completed school. Elana asked me to help her with her classes while she went on maternity leave. She and I worked together as partners for over ten years. She had birthed yoga at the college and had a strong program going. She trusted me enough to assist her and it meant the world to me. Together, we built the yoga program to four classes a week and over eighty students per semester over those ten years. The two of us would team teach over a thousand students in the time we were together. I began getting calls and requests to teach in health clubs, studios, workshops, and events. This continued from 2001 to 2011.

In 2008, I opened my school with the blessing of my teachers and as of the publication of this book in fall 2017, Balance Yoga and Wellness has trained nearly two hundred students to teach. From 2012 to 2014 I had a studio. When management changed and my rent increased substantially, I decided the time was right for me to let go of the studio and work as a traveling teacher, which I had always enjoyed more than owning a brick and mortar business.

Not a day goes by that I go to bed feeling like an expert. Every day, I wake feeling like there is a sea of information in this world that I need to learn. I am now working in the medical field in lifestyle medicine as a yoga therapist, teaching various trainings, and have been hard at work on this book for some time. I wear many hats. It's been a great career, but one of very hard work, some tough lessons, and one that asks a lot of me on many levels repeatedly. This field is not for the faint of heart—you must work hard, study, and constantly deal with your ego as it will be reflected to you on a regular basis. It is joyful work, it is good work, but it is work nonetheless and one must be able to get up, show up, and give back on a regular basis. One tough part is that not everyone will like you. Anytime you put yourself out there, some people will love you and some people will be jealous and some people will just plain not care for what you offer. This is why I find it so important to reiterate to my students the importance of self care, having their own practices, and maintaining a loving and supportive network of people they can talk to.

Learning Styles

Students learn in a variety of ways, including watching you do or orchestrate a pose with your hands (visual), through listening to your words (auditory), and/or through experiencing or doing a pose (kinesthetic). All three are valuable. It is important to remember that much like a game of Simon Says, if you only model poses people will try to emulate you and could get hurt. Though visual cueing is valuable, a class should have a good balance of all three. It is also very important to get up and walk the room, to guide the students with your words, your hands, and by allowing them to experience the postures for themselves.

Walking the Room for Safety

Personally, I find my classes work best if I am in front of the room in the beginning of class when students (especially new students) are facing the front. Then as I take them to all fours (hands and knees), and into sun salutations, etc., I am more likely to be walking the room. It is important to tell new students what to expect, so let them know that throughout the class you may leave your mat and walk the room. You should aim to be off your mat about 50% of the class time. Once you are comfortable, you may find you are off your mat 2/3 of the time or more. That said, in my work in lifestyle medicine I do not walk the room. In this teaching role, my students often are ill or have hearing issues, so I am in front of them most of the time unless I am assisting them to be more comfortable or to get into a posture. It is important for all students to learn to be independent, so do only as much as is needed for them.

It is very important that to watch and adjust students for safety, and not to be afraid to help them to be safe, whether that help is verbal or manual.

Teaching Tips:
Verbal Cuing

Before leaving the mat to walk the room, provide a cue like, *"Hold your posture while inhaling and exhaling."* This language allows the student to know not to emulate or move from the posture as the teacher departs the mat. You might also mention at the beginning or during class that you may help them with adjustments for safety or even to deepen a pose if they are ready. Realize that some students will believe they are doing the pose "wrong" and may feel embarrassed, so it is important to make them feel comfortable and use permissive language. Verbal help might include words spoken softly directly to an individual student or noting something to the entire class. For example, *"If this posture is uncomfortable, try softening the knees or elbows and see how that feels."* Such directions may allow the student to make the adjustment on their own and to recognize how to self-check their alignment next time.

Hands-on Adjustments

My hands-on assisting is often done when students are looking down or away (twists and forward folds), or when they are holding a pose for a few rounds of breath (like Warrior 1). This allows space for personal boundaries to be maintained as teacher and student become familiar with each other. New teachers can start with gently adjusting students in child's pose, down dog, and Shavasana until they are more comfortable with assisting. If for some reason a teacher is not comfortable with assisting whatsoever, be prepared with strong verbal cues.

Identifying Community Needs

Take special note of your clients and the people in your community by considering their needs and desires. You may be in an urban area that has fit young executives, which may lead you to assume they all want a hard-core, power yoga class. They might, but they may also be looking for a way to relax and rejuvenate. In that case, you may want to offer both options. Or you may be in a retirement community and need to offer more therapeutic-based classes using chairs. Pay attention, be sensitive to students' needs, and prepare to be flexible. You may go into teaching believing you will be the next power yoga teacher only to be thrown into subbing a gentle class. You may find that you quite love what you didn't think you would! I have had many teacher-students of mine come to me with this experience. Be open.

Section 4: Physical and Energetic Anatomy

When most people think of anatomy, the systems of the physical body come most readily to mind. In yoga, the physical and energetic anatomy work hand-in-hand to sustain life and drive its processes. The life force energy known by yogis as prana (which you'll learn more about in Section 5) is the foundation of life and indeed, of the whole universe. This vital energy courses through our bodies, initiating all actions from physical movements to biochemical processes.

Physical Anatomy/Systems of the Human Body

For this portion of the *Guide*, I recommend deepening understanding by pairing the contents of this section with more expansive anatomy books. These may include books like Leslie Kaminoff's *Yoga Anatomy*, any of Ray Long's many anatomy books, or others. There are also many online resources.

- **Circulatory** — heart, blood vessels, blood, lymphatic system, lymphatic vessels, and lymph.

- **Digestive** — mouth, pharynx, esophagus, stomach, small and large intestines, accessory organs such as gallbladder and pancreas.

- **Endocrine** — includes all the glands of the body and the hormones produced by those glands, including the pituitary, thyroid, parathyroid, adrenal, thymus, and pineal glands, as well as the hypothalamus, pancreas, ovaries, and testes.

- **Integumentary** — skin, hair, nails, glands.

- **Muscular** — skeletal, smooth, and cardiac muscles.

- **Nervous** — brain, spinal cord, and all peripheral nerves.

- **Reproductive** — sex organs.

- **Respiratory** — mouth, nasal cavity, bronchia, trachea, pharynx, lungs and lobes, ribs.

- **Skeletal** — bones, joints, cartilage, and connective tissue.

- **Special Sense System** — eyes, ears, nose, and taste buds.

- **Urinary** — kidneys, ureters, bladder, and urethra.

Circulatory System

The circulatory system is comprised of the cardiovascular and lymphatic systems, which circulate and distribute blood and lymph. Yoga assists in increasing circulation in the body, which provides rejuvenation of the blood through increased oxygen. When the heart contracts it sends blood to the lungs where it picks up oxygen and carries it to all the cells of the body.

Through pranayama and movement (through asana), the blood vessels and arteries are kept more elastic. This is beneficial for contraction and expansion, allowing for increased blood flow. The practice assists in calming the nervous system which helps to regulate blood pressure, heart rate, and cortisol levels which have a direct correlation with plaque that leads to cardiovascular disease. Lymph fluid is moved through the body with pranayama and asana, helping to avoid lymphatic congestion which can cause a variety of problems. Movement helps lymph to move and allows the white blood cells to properly do their job of healing. Healthy circulation and movement of the circulatory and lymph system equal a healthier person.

Digestive System

The digestive system carries nutrients to our body and is responsible for getting rid of waste products. It is comprised of the mouth, pharynx, esophagus, stomach, small and large intestines, and accessory organs such as the gallbladder and pancreas. Yoga helps to keep our digestive system balanced through asana and massage of our internal organs. Meditation is helpful for stress-related digestive problems.

Endocrine System

The endocrine system includes all the glands of the body and the hormones produced by those glands. It includes the pituitary, thyroid, parathyroid, adrenal, thymus, and pineal glands, as well as the hypothalamus, pancreas, ovaries, and testes. Amazingly, the endocrine system lines up perfectly in the body with the chakra system developed many thousands of years ago. Yoga practices have a direct impact on the stress response for which endocrine system is responsible through the production of hormones.

Cortisol is a hormone often talked about, and has been linked to fat accumulation in the body. When reducing stress, one in turn reduces the body's need to produce cortisol. Less cortisol production can lead to increased melatonin production, melatonin production being responsible for controlling sleep and wake cycles.

Poses like cobra and upward-facing dog (which are backbends) can massage and stimulate the thymus, helping to increase immunity to illness.

Integumentary System

The integumentary system includes skin, hair, nails, and glands. Our body gets rid of waste material though respiration, perspiration, and elimination.

When we breathe shallowly, we are not getting enough oxygen to our organs, including our skin. When we fail to fully exhale we leave carbon dioxide in the recesses of our lungs, which is also taxing to our brains. Full inhalations and exhalations remove waste products from our bodies, allowing our skin, hair, and nails to be healthier and more vibrant.

Sweating is a natural way of detoxifying the body and getting waste products out through the pores. Stress reduction may also help prevent breakouts and skin reactions. The ancient practice of dry brushing and exfoliation is part of a healthy yoga practice as well.

Muscular System

The muscular system produces movement in the body in conjunction with the joints, and stabilizes and supports the body. Muscles contract and extend, sending messages to the brain through the nervous system.

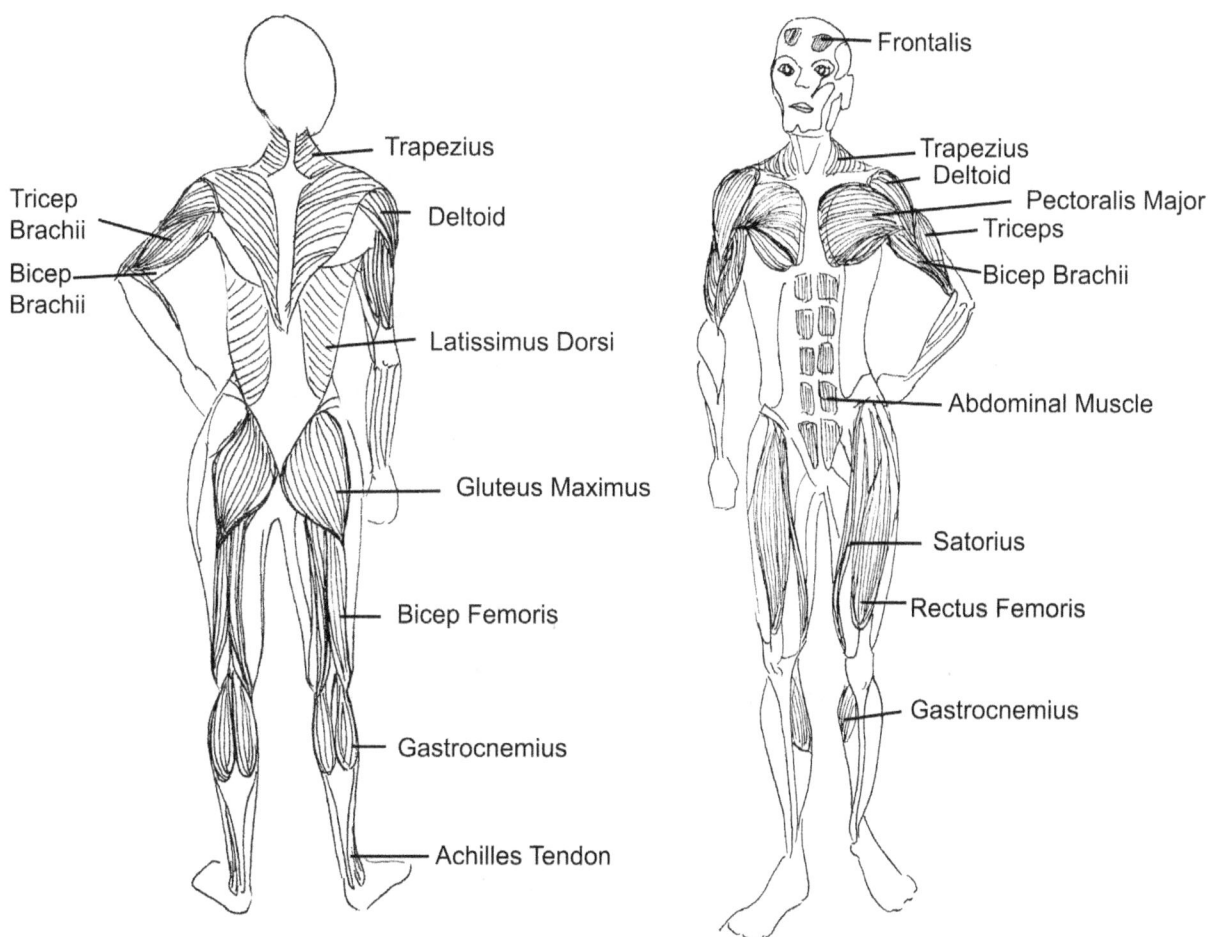

In yoga, for every contraction (shortening) of one muscle there is be extension (lengthening) of the opposite muscle. This is a very important point in understanding the concept of balance in the body. If you contract the front thighs (quadriceps), you are extending the back thighs (hamstrings). Yoga asanas should always balance each muscle. For instance, if you do a backbend lengthening the front body, you will counter with a forward bend lengthening the back body. When you are discussing the torso, you can also counter with a twist. One example would be when you do a forward cobbler pose, you could raise and twist to lengthen the sides of the front torso or a backbend to do the same. Twists counter backbends and forward folds, which is important to note when sequencing a class.

Through pranayama and asana, which you'll learn about in the next section, the muscles are massaged and blood flow is increased. Collagen is maintained in the tissues, and muscle tone is maintained and built. The major muscle groups are massaged, including the heart muscle by bringing healthy blood flow to and from the heart.

Nervous System

The nervous system includes the brain, spinal cord, and all peripheral nerves. These organs work together to control and regulate the body, and facilitate communication among its parts.

Pranayama, asana and meditation all have a profound effect on our nervous system. In times of stress we go into a flight or fight response. It is said that our body often goes through this response several times a day in stressful situations. Learning to properly breathe brings oxygen to the body and calms the nervous system. The postures play a big part in calming the nervous system, as well. Certain poses, like forward bend, put pressure on the frontal lobes of the brain where our reasoning and analytical thinking are located. Forward folds also massage the parasympathetic nerve in the low back and neck allowing the body mind to relax. Forward poses massage and calm this part of the brain, activating a calming response in the body. Many studies have shown that mediation helps strengthen and thicken the brain in areas that are responsible for the flight or fight response. This is one reason many forward thinking hospitals like Scripps Hospitals are now utilizing yoga for their patients. When the nervous system is under control, the patient is able to better control and manage their pain.

Reproductive System

The reproductive system is made up of the sex organs. The medical community is generally of the consensus that yoga is good for infertility, menstrual pain, and symptoms of menopause. Men benefit as well, as yoga postures bring increase blood flow and oxygen to the organs in the groin and pelvis.

Women are often able to reduce menstrual pain with yoga poses that relax the abdomen (like cobbler), and with other yoga-inspired relaxation techniques. Menopausal women are often able to reduce hot flashes through relaxation. Studies show that stress plays a great factor in infertility for some women and men. Relaxation can help males produce more sperm through increased circulation and regulation of the nervous system. In females, it is less clear how relaxation impacts fertility. However, we do know that blood volume is increased greatly through the practice of yoga—especially in poses like legs up the wall and inversions that bring blood flow to the sex organs—which deliver fresh oxygen via blood to the sex organs and carry away waste products through increased circulation.

Personal Story:
Yoga and Fertility

My teacher Elana came to yoga because she heard it was good for infertility. She had one child and was having trouble getting pregnant again. Four kids later, she is a great testament to the theory of yoga's impact on fertility. In my own school, Balance Yoga and Wellness, we have had many women get pregnant during training—about 10%!

Respiratory System

The respiratory system includes the mouth, nasal cavity, bronchia, trachea, pharynx, lungs and lobes, and ribs.

Without breath there is no life. Pranayama provides breathing practices that teach one to fully inhale oxygen and fully exhale carbon dioxide, increasing lung capacity and the life and health of the lungs. Breathwork helps to regulate our nervous system, our blood pressure, and our heart rate. This practice has an overall calming effect on the body which in turn creates healing as our stress hormones are regulated. When we inhale we take in oxygen: when we exhale we expel carbon dioxide and oxygen is pushed into the blood stream as we exhale. Full diaphragmatic breathing helps to keep the ribs and spine from stiffening with age. The intercostal muscles are expanded and stretched with each breath. Those with asthma and COPD often find great improvement in their breathing when they practice deep breathing.

Personal Story:
Pranayama and Asthma

During my childhood, I developed serious lung damage due to years of exposure to secondhand smoke. At age 29, I was struggling with serious asthma attacks that landed me in the ER more than once. With proper diagnosis, which included allergy shots, I did improve some, but still suffered with shortness of breath. Though I was a practicing yogi I was not giving full attention to the breath. I increased my pranayama practice and have not had to use an inhaler more than a few times in the past fifteen years. I credit this to the breathwork.

Skeletal System

The skeletal system creates the framework for the structure of the body, including the muscles and the fascia. It protects the heart, lungs, and brain. It also serves as a lever system to allow for movement through muscular contraction. Bones store minerals and produce red blood cells. Bones are alive and carry out many important functions. The skeletal system is like the alignment on a car. Asana helps to maintain healthy structural alignment through movement. Many postures are weight-bearing and help to increase the density and strength of bones.

Caution:
Fall and Injury Risks

If a person has osteopenia or osteoporosis, one should always be careful when practicing to avoid falls. A chair, a bar, or props can be used to reduce the chance of falling. It is always best to practice poses that are not a fall risk. Deep twists are also to be modified with osteopenia and osteoporosis to avoid the possibility of fractures in the spine. Also, a word about the cervical spine and inversions. The neck is made to hold 8 lbs of head (not 100+ pounds of body). Headstands, handstands, and many of the more challenging inversions are considered advanced asanas, and should only be done by students who have ample experience and are guided by a teacher. As a teacher, I do not recommend teaching headstands or handstands in beginner or intermediate classes.

Joints

There are six types of joints:
1. **Gliding** — fingers
2. **Hinge** — knees and elbows
3. **Ball and Socket** — hips and shoulders
4. **Saddle** — thumbs
5. **Condyloid or Ellipsoidal** — convex surfaces like the wrist
6. **Pivot** — vertebra

The roles of cartilage, collagen, tendons, ligaments, synovial fluid, and fascia:

- **Cartilage** serves as the soft tissue that prevents our bones from clanking or rubbing together.

- **Collagen** is the body's most abundant protein and is the substance that holds the body together.

- **Tendons** connect muscle to bone.

- **Ligaments** connect bone to bone.

- **Fascia** separates as well as connects everything in the body. It is like a stocking over the body holding everything together.

- **Synovial Fluid** is the fluid inside synovial joints. Synovial fluid has a calming effect on the body and reduces friction during movement. (Poses that massage the large ball and socket joints such as the hips and shoulders offer a calming effect as they massage the synovial fluid in the joint.)

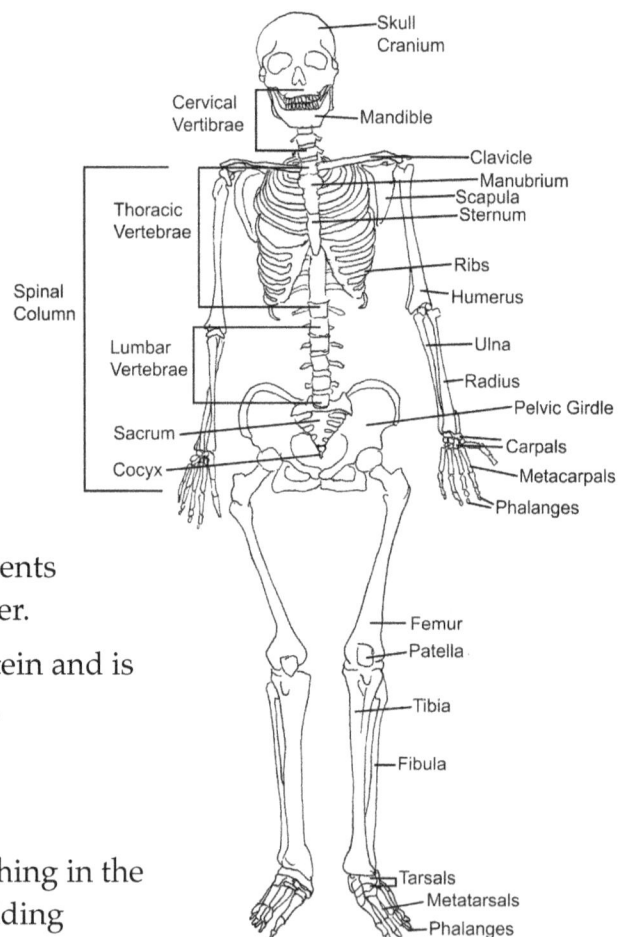

Special Sense System

Includes the eyes, ears, nose, and taste buds.

Utilizing your senses and sense withdrawal falls under limb number five. I teach withdrawal by first asking students to engage one sense and shut out all others. For example, one might listen with the ears while shutting out the senses of sight, touch, taste, and smell. Then, one might let their hearing go and focus on vision and so on. This practice builds not only inner perceptual awareness but a heightened sense of enjoyment from being in the moment. It allows us to fully resonate with everything going on around us, and also to withdraw and cope with life when things are hectic. This practice is helpful in pain management, stress management, and learning to listen to our inner voices. It decreases the likelihood of dangerous behaviors like overeating or substance abuse due to emotional stress. Through it, one can learn to distinguish between what is actually happening on the physical level versus a psychological level.

Personal Story:
MRI and Sensory Withdrawl
Once, when I was getting a brain MRI, I found myself on the verge of panic. The sounds were simply awful and I was scared in the MRI hole. I called on my meditation skills and ability to withdraw my senses to go to a place in my mind that was relaxing. It is comforting to know I can rely on this practice wherever and whenever I need it.

Urinary System

Includes kidneys, ureters, bladder, and urethra. Yoga asana squeezes and massages our internal organs, bringing fresh blood flow to the urinary system and helping assist movement of waste out of the body.

Energetic Anatomy

Energetic anatomy often brings about confusion in the new yogi, and can take much study to make sense. Though Eastern medicine and philosophy have provided time-tested practices to improve health and wellbeing, Westerners are often skeptical about energetic anatomy. Western Medicine tends to deal with the person on a physical anatomical level while Eastern Medicine takes a more holistic approach. The West is catching up with a rise in the number of integrative physicians and naturopaths, and more integrative therapies being recognized by insurance companies as well as in hospitals and clinics.

As noted throughout this book, the vastness of yoga would take many lifetimes to learn. I've offered a basic overview of energetic anatomy here, but encourage further study based on your curiosities. In the practice of yoga therapy, we often go much deeper. It is my hope that this will be a simple guide to assist you in expanding your understanding of yoga practices and how they relate to a person on a holistic level.

Yoga is like a quilt of many fabrics. The lineage comes from the East, but not just from one area. For me, letting go of having to put these categories and their components in chronological order helped me learn more about energetic anatomy. Understanding energetic anatomy is much like looking at a hologram. It is not static or flat, is not linear, and has layers of influences from many religions, disciplines, and geographical locations. Any "side" from which you view it will offer a different vision and a varied perspective.

Ayurveda

Some would say yoga derives from Ayurveda (the science of life still practiced in India and around the world today), and some would say it's a sister science. From all my study, I would say all that we really know is that they are related. In the study of Ayurveda, yoga and yogic principles are used to heal ailments ranging from psychological distress to physical pain and beyond. If you were to travel to an Ayurvedic hospital in India, you would undergo a series of treatments usually lasting for several weeks called panchakarma. Panchakarma has many layers, including yoga; oil rubbing; cleansing through diet, meditation, and contemplation; and other specific treatments. The practices have had great results over thousands of years. Though you may not go to an Ayurvedic hospital any time soon, you can bring many of these practices into your daily life to improve overall health and wellbeing.

An Approach from Early Childhood Education

By education, I am a teacher of children and so I often like to take hard subjects and imagine I am explaining them to children. I've found that if you can teach something to a child then you can learn it on a much deeper level, in part because it is difficult to understand the nuance before you grasp a root understanding. Take what you can, but do not stress if you don't understand it all. I have been studying and practicing yoga for two-thirds of my life, yet I know I have miles to go and lifetimes of study would be needed for me to grasp every concept of this ancient science. I'll share a very basic working knowledge of the energetic anatomy, derived from my years of practice and self-study.

Let me explain energetic anatomy as I might to a private yoga therapy client. You are familiar with the nervous system, right? That includes your nerves, your spinal column, and your brain. This is the method of sending signals throughout your body. In yoga, we talk about a signal system called nadis that lines up closely with the nerves in the body, and chakras that line up with the spine and brain. Tantra yoga indicates that we have over 72,000 nadis, 108 of which are said to be of great importance. Nadis are points in the body. Much like acupressure or acupuncture releases blockages in the body (in Ayurveda we call this ama), so too does the practice of yoga. Through pranayama, asana, meditation, diet, and living by the yamas and niyamas, we experience release and relief. Another interesting fact is that the chakras also line up with the endocrine system, the spine and the brain.

When thinking of nadis, consider them as pathways of energy. These can and do get blocked with ama, a sticky substance that can be represented in the West by things like cholesterol, tumors, cysts, or simple emotional blockages and pain. It is so important here to avoid using this thinking to feel shameful or to shame others. We all have stress and pain in our lives from illnesses and other events beyond our control. If one gets cancer, we do not blame the person. The cancer could stem from something environmental or genetic.

Nadis

Nadis encompass all the points in the body through which energy flows to the chakras. Nadi derives from the root "nad," which is Sanskrit for "flow" or "motion." There are believed to be over 72,000 nadis, 108 of which are of importance in the yogic world. Some say meridians, nadis, and chakras are the same, while others believe they are like three corresponding flowing energies that exist separately but follow the same pathways. These paths can get stuck or blocked and yoga practices can assist in clearing them.

The three nadis of greatest importance are the ida, pingala, and sushumna. Think of the ida and the pingala nadis as a double helix going up the spine, surrounding the sushumna ("most gracious") nadi.

- **Ida** — Left side of the body, connecting with the left nostril. Cool, dark, dense, moon, passive, more of a yin quality. The ida controls mental processes.

- **Pingala** — Right side of the body, connecting with right nostril. Light, warm, airy, active, sun, more of a yang quality. The pingala controls vital processes.

- **Sushumna** — The primary nadi that goes up the spine, passing through each of the seven chakras. The ida and pingala double helix around it. The sushumna is the pathway to heightened consciousness or spiritual awakening.

Ama

Ama is anything that is a blockage or a toxin in our body. It is often referred to as a sticky substance such as cholesterol or tumors that occur in our bodies, but there are other types of ama as well. Often environmental factors, stress, diet, and lack of healthy habits lead to illness in the body. When I or another yoga teacher or medical professional says, *"The issues are stored in our tissues"* this is one of the *issues* we are speaking of. I often explain this as "dis-ease leads to disease." I believe strongly though that there are many type of issues we store and not all can be seen with the naked eye or with technological medical tools.

Samskaras

Samskaras are habits that get stored in our bodies, our muscle memories, and our minds. They are often referred to as impressions formed in the mind. For instance, we may have the habit of negative thinking or the habit of buying bananas every time we go to the store. These patterns are stored in our minds and in our bodies. In yogic philosophy, it is often the patterns we retain from this life and past lives. Samskaras are not necessarily negative; they can be healthy habits as well. I personally think of them as the pathways our brains develop from what we learn. Samskaras are not inevitable or irreversible. For example, we may have grown up with unhealthy eating habits; it takes work, but we can change those patterns.

Koshas and Doshas

Koshas

In Ayurvedic science koshas and doshas guide us in our understanding of ourselves and others. Koshas are the facets or levels of the human body. Doshas are the archetypes of the human body related to the five elements.

Koshas include the five facets of the human being:

1. **Annamayakosha** — The physical body, as nourished by food. The form, solid structure, and balance of the body through all five elements: earth, water, fire, air, and space.

2. **Pranamayakosha** — The energy body, including chakras and energy channels. The intake and flow of prana (life force) in the body.

3. **Manomayakosha** — The psycho-emotional body. Drives and emotional responses such as fight or flight. Blockages from stress can manifest into physical or mental illness.

4. **Vijnyanamayakosha** — Wisdom body. Wisdom, intuition, insight. The witness observer that recognizes life patterns and how to change them.

5. **Anandamayakosha** — Bliss body. The true self is one of inner contentment and connection to the divine or that of a greater understanding than what is tangible on this earth.

Doshas

The three doshas—Vata, Pitta, and Kapha—are mind-body types into which every human is said to fall. Each dosha expresses a unique combination of physical, emotional, and mental characteristics, and is derived from the five elements.

Doshas

1. **Vata** — Combines air and space. Person tends to be light in structure. Usually taller or petite and thinner. Vata types are creative, subtle, and full of new ideas.

2. **Pitta** — Mostly fire with some water. Pittas tend to have a medium build and are more muscular. Generally friendly, outgoing, strong, brave.

3. **Kapha** — Earth and water. Kaphas remind me of turtles. They are heavier in build and have larger frames, move slower, and are gentle in nature.

<u>The Five Elements</u>

All living things, including our bodies, are made up of these five elements that are the building blocks of all matter:

- **Earth** — Heavy, dense, solid, plants, the earth, animals. First chakra (root) and annamayakosha.

- **Water** — Liquid, flowing, penetrating. Second chakra (sacral) and pranamayakosha.

- **Fire** — Sun, heat, energy. Third chakra (solar plexus) and manomayakosha.

- **Air** — Breath, oxygen, gases. Fourth chakra (heart) and vijnyanamayakosha.

- **Space** — Mobile, spirit, ambient. Fifth (throat), sixth (third eye), and seventh (crown) chakras, anandamayakosha.

We all would do well to strive on a daily basis for a balanced life. This includes tending to all areas of our life. People have to tend to their physical health through diet, exercise, proper relaxation, meditation, sleep, and positive thinking. I would also add that getting out in nature is essential for balancing the doshas. For instance, when you are feeling ungrounded, try digging in the dirt or standing with your feet in the grass. Sometimes I will simply go outside and touch the ground or a tree as the Buddhist monks do to connect with nature and life.

We don't have to fully understand all of these concepts to benefit from engaging with them. If you will just notice what makes you feel calm, at peace, and whole, then you know intuitively what you need to balance your doshas, chakras, and koshas. It is really as simple as paying attention to the patterns in your life, your preferences, your likes and dislikes.

Personal Story:
The Call of Water
Not until later in life did I realize I was a pitta dosha and that I need water to calm my fiery nature that is often full of anxiety. When I moved to Houston, I felt a desperate need to be back near the lakes, mountains, and hardwoods of my home in Arkansas. My heart and soul literally ached for these outdoor elements to the point that every three weeks I drove eight hours home to see my family and to be back in nature.

The Chakras

Chakra means "wheel," and the chakras are centers in the body through which energy flows. Most are familiar with 7 chakras, but there are actually 114 wheels in the body that relate to us on many different levels and produce different qualities in us. In addition to the nadis, these are the channels along which vital energy ("prana") moves. An easy way to remember the color of the chakras is that they are the same as a rainbow: red, orange, yellow, green, blue, indigo and violet, so you can use the acronym ROYGBIV.

In yoga we often think of postures as the balancing forces for the chakras and they do assist in balancing the chakras along with other practices like breathing, meditation, and many other activities. The postures are ideal vehicles through which one can begin to achieve balance in the body mind. Over time, the introduction of the knowledge of chakras and other facets of the energetic body begin to aid in balance as well.

This is the beauty and wisdom of this ancient practice.

First Chakra — Muladhara
Location: Perineal floor
Element: Earth
Color: Red
Function: Survival
Verb: I have
Affirmation: To be here
Shadow Emotions: Resistance, rigidity, resentment
Impact: Kidneys, eliminatory systems, feet, legs, spine, joints
Postures: Standing poses, seated forward folds, boat, seated twist, grounding postures
Kosha: Annamayakosha

Second Chakra — Svadhisthana
Location: Four fingers below navel, sex organs
Element: water
Color: orange
Function: Sexuality
Verb: I feel
Affirmation: To feel
Shadow Emotions: Desire, passion, manipulation, greed
Impact: Reproductive system
Postures: Cobbler, hero, reverse table, hip openers, camel, arm balances
Koshas: Pranamayakosha

Third Chakra — Manipura

Location: Naval center to solar plexus
Element: Fire
Color: Yellow
Function: Personal power, self, ego
Verb: I can
Affirmation: To act
Shadow Emotions: Insecurity, anger, greed, low self-esteem
Impact : Stomach, liver, gallbladder, digestion
Postures: Twists, locust, bow, child's pose, pyramid, cobra, backbends
Koshas: Manomayakosha

Fourth Chakra — Anahata

Location: Heart
Element: Air
Color: Green
Function: Love
Verb: I love
Affirmation: To love
Shadow Emotions: Fear, attachment
Impact: Circulation, heart
Postures: Backbends, lateral bends, cobra, child's pose, bridge, tree, warrior 2, camel
Kosha: Manomayakosha and Vijnyanamayakosha

Fifth Chakra — Vishuddha

Location: Throat
Element: Ether
Color: Blue
Function: Intuition, communication
Verb: I speak
Affirmation: To speak
Shadow Emotions: Inability to speak, denial, gossip
Impact: Lungs, throat, ears
Postures: Shoulder stand, twists, cobra, up dog, forward bends
Kosha: Vijnyanamayakosha

Sixth Chakra — Ajna

Location: Third Eye
Element: all elements
Color: Indigo
Function: Intuition, mind
Verb: I see

Affirmation: To see
Shadow Emotions: Confusion, expression, lack of integration of intuition into life
Impact: Lower brain, eyes, nose, the senses
Postures: Balance poses, child's pose, rabbit, forward bends, down dog
Kosha: Anandamayakosha

Seventh Chakra — Sahasrara

Location: Crown of head
Element: beyond color, crystal light, time and space.
Color: Violet or beyond color crystal light
Function: Knowing, oneness
Verb: I know
Affirmation: To know
Shadow Emotions: Grief, depression
Impact: Upper brain and nervous system
Postures: Inversions, lotus, down dog
Kosha: Anandamayakosha

Eighth Chakra — The Radiance, The Aura

The eighth chakra is said to be the gateway to the true, higher self and/or to the divine. This level of energy work is best saved for advanced yoga studies.

Energy Anatomy

COLOR	CHAKRA 8: Aura	ELEMENT	DOSHA	KOSHA	BANDHA	IMPACT ON ENDOCRINE SYSTEM AND HEALTH	GUNAS
Violet	7: Sahasrara/ Crown Chakra	Crystal Light		Anandamayakosha		*Pineal* Separation from source	Energies in nature, including in the human mind.
Indigo	6: Ajna/ Third Eye Chakra	All		Anandamayakosha	Jalandhara Bandha	*Pituitary* Senses	<u>Rajas</u> Desire
Blue	5: Vishuddha/ Throat Chakra	Space	Vatta	Vijnyanamayakosha		*Thyroid and Para-Thyroid* Speech	Active Attachment Fight or Flight: Run
Green	4: Anahata/ Heart Chakra	Air	Vatta	Vijnyanamayakosha Manomayakosha	Uddiyana Bandha	*Thymus* Respiratory, Heart	<u>Sattva:</u> Balance Clarity Light
Yellow	3: Manipura/ Solar Plexus Chakra	Fire	Pitta	Manomayakosha		*Pancreas, Adrenals Stomach, Liver, Small Intestine*	<u>Tamas:</u> Apathy Stuck
Orange	2: Svadhisthana/ Naval Chakra (4 Fingers Below Naval)	Water	Pitta Kapha	Pranamayakosha	Mula Bandha	*Ovaries* Reproduction, Pelvic Area	Inertia
Red	1: Muladhara/ Root Chakra	Earth	Kapha	Annamayakosha		*Testicles* Elimination, Legs/Feet	Fight or Flight: Freeze

Personal Stories:

Balancing the Chakras

I personally deal with a lot of digestive and thyroid issues. As a child, my needs were simply not being met. My early life was full of pain from divorce, being moved around from house to house, family addiction, and more. As I grew up, I was in a string of abusive relationships. In the past, when I experienced stomach or low belly issues, I would curl up in a ball up on the bed or in the bathtub from the pain. Later in life, I figured out that I have blockages, pain, and disease processes in my root, throat, and sacral chakras. Now I have realized better coping skills, including walking in nature, doing a series of balanced postures that target those areas, and meditation. Without fail, with the help of my practice, I always get relief. It is not perfect, but my condition always improves, even if it is only temporary. Practice is not a cure, but a set of tools to gain the self-awareness that can assist us as we continually work to bring ourselves into balance.

Throat Chakra

My favorite colors are turquoise and red. The throat chakra color is turquoise and the lower root is red. I have been decorating with these colors for many years. When I was 23 I had two thirds of my thyroid removed and have been on thyroid related medicine since then. My tendencies have always been to please others first, to not speak my mind, and to worry about others' feelings to the point of suffering myself. Now I know that certain practices help me to open and balance this chakra. Examples include drinking peppermint tea, saying my affirmations, meditating on opening my throat, letting sun and air into a window, and doing poses that open that area, such as fish pose. These practices help me to feel more open and able to express myself in a healthy way.

Mantras, Mudras, and Bandhas

Mantras, Mudras, and Bandhas are ancient healing arts.

Mantra — A hymn, phrase, or word repeated to bring us higher consciousness and awareness much the same way as an affirmation. You may wish to learn more about the mantras associated with each chakra.

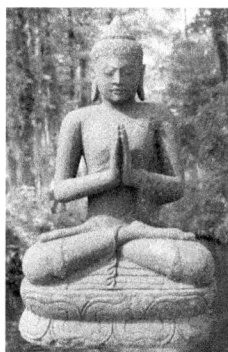

Mudra — Hand gestures that are said to influence the flow of energy in the body. For example, a "lotus mudra" should help one feel grounded and strong, opening toward joy and light.

Anjali mudra (hands placed together at the center of the chest) is often done at the end of class following shavasana, symbolizing sealing the practice. Anjali mudra is the gesture associated with the Sanskrit salutation, Namaste, and is often performed as the student says, "Namaste," a mantra which means *"The love and light in me, or my highest self, recognizes the love and light in you or your highest self."* After anjali mudra, the student may bow as a symbol of mutual respect or to seal the practice and mark the ending and yet a new beginning.

Bandhas — Locks, the purpose of which is to control energy in the body. Some teachers believe that these should only be taught to advanced students, but it is common to hear teachers talk about bandhas. There four main bandhas.

1. *Mula Bandha* — Lift and contract your pelvic floor muscles. Pull the muscles as if you are stopping your urine stream.

2. *Uddiyana Bandha* — Lifting of the diaphragm. My teacher explained it as lifting the muscles you use when you vomit. You can teach yourself to hold this bandha and exhale and inhale but this often takes many years of practice. Therefore it is not used as much in common hatha yoga classes.

3. *Jalandhara Bandha* — There are two form of this chin lock. One is to take the chin and rest it in the soft spot in the low neck below the thyroid. The other and the easier one is to hold the head erect over the torso, put a flat hand up to your nose, and pull back one inch. This should slightly lower the chin.

4. *Maha Bandha* — When all three bandhas are done at once.

Terms in vogue in the yoga world which are more for instructional purposes but are sometimes referred to as bandhas include:

Hasta Bandha — "Hand Lock" — This is becoming a common way to explain mindful hand positioning for down dog and other poses with hands on the floor. Hands generally will be facing the front of the mat and parallel to one another. Thumb and forefinger will be pressed down as well as the pads of the fingers, while a slight suction cup is made with the middle of the palm.

Pada Bandha — "Foot Lock" — This term is being used to describe mindful foot positioning in standing poses and poses with the sole of the foot on the floor. Feet should be flat pressing through the toe pads, ball of the foot pressing down, little toe side of the foot pressing down, and heel pressing down, with arches lifted. I teach this as pressing down as if you are connecting four tires on a car into the earth. I have also heard it taught as a tripod, connect your foot like a tripod to the earth.

RAJAS	SATTVA	TAMAS
Anxiety	Balance	Lethargy
Selfishness		Apathy
Desire	Clarity	Stuck
Active	Positivity	Inertia
Attachment		Fight or Flight: Freeze
Fight or Flight: Run	Light	

Gunas

The Gunas reflect the ever-changing energies in nature. Practicing yoga brings one to a Sattvic state, or a state of balance. Simply put, by practicing a yogic or a healthy lifestyle one can achieve balance, or at the very least hold the necessary tools to bring themselves back into balance. When one gets overly active or overexcited, one is in a Rajastic state. When one is depressed or low on energy, one is in a Tamastic state.

Basics of Energetic Anatomy

Understanding energetic anatomy is a lot to absorb and develops over time. Your yoga practice should always include pranayama and postures that are balanced, moving the spine in all six directions, such as forward bends, backbends, lateral side leans to the left and right, and twists to the left and right. Add inversions to bring it all to a higher level, and then add meditation to complete the process.

In your daily life, follow a healthy lifestyle of moderation. Live an ethical and moral life making good decisions. Care for yourself by eating healthfully, exercising regularly, and getting enough sleep. Surround yourself with positive people and stimuli. Avoid negativity in your life. Meditate regularly, even for short periods, remembering that any effort is better than none. Get out and enjoy nature at least once a day, touch the earth, swim, look at the stars and the moon and the sky. You do not have to be an expert in energetic anatomy to understand that this practice, which is a lifestyle, offers balance, connection, and contentment that will bring a deep happiness to your life.

> *Teaching Tip:*
> **Bringing Energy into Balance**
> When I practice asana, I often think about how the postures are moving energy via my blood volume and nervous system through my chakras. It is incredible to think that when this system originated, the ancients so intuitively understood the human systems of the body and how they worked: the functions of the physical and emotional bodies truly do line up with the functions of the energetic body. Amazing!

The postures and practices experienced in a well-taught, basic hatha yoga class bring balance to the koshas, the doshas, the gunas, and the chakras, as well as assist in changing patterns and behaviors and removing blockages leaving the student more holistically aligned. Have you yourself experienced or have you had a student experience this? Say a student begins taking yoga classes, believing they are just exercising and relaxing. However, over time they start to notice changes not just in their body but in their behavior. Possibly they notice they feel more patient and at ease. This is the example I hear most often. I also hear that people say they reduce their need to overindulge in unhealthy behaviors because they reduce the stress that caused the desire for these substances or habits.

If we practice, remain curious, and continue to inquire, its pretty remarkable how yoga can shape our lives.

Section 5: Limbs 3 and 4, Pranayama and Asana

Pranayama

Pranayama practice includes breathing methods that assist in bringing "prana" into the body and controlling the flow of prana, or "life force." This thing we call prana is not only breath—it is what enters our bodies upon our first breath and what leaves us upon our death, when life itself enters and exits our bodies. Different types of pranayama practices have varying functions; however, all bring balance to the body.

When we breathe in oxygen, we are bringing a life-giving substance into our body that we must have to live. When we exhale carbon dioxide, we are expelling what we don't need and is toxic to our bodies. Without each process, we would die. Also when we exhale, plants and trees turn our carbon dioxide into oxygen and give it back to us. Without them we would not survive. This recognition furthers our connection to the world around us.

Prana is the movement of not just oxygen, but also energy in the body. When a person practices breathing techniques, the benefits are huge. The heart is massaged, the spine is lengthened, the intercostal muscles are stretched, and the lungs are exercised all with the expansion and contraction of breath. At the same time the nervous system is bought under control. With properly practiced pranayama, the body goes into a parasympathetic state, relaxing and renewing the body mind, reducing cortisol (stress hormones), and bringing the body out of flight, fight, or collapse and into homeostasis or balance.

When we don't breathe properly all kinds of dis-ease sets in. Of course, centuries ago, there were no X-Rays or CT Scans to see inside our bodies. But even before the ability to peek inside living bodies through these technologies, people realized something amazing was going on and gave it a name. Mystics and wise people knew that on a holistic level we need balance and understood that one of the key ways to be balanced is through our breath.

When we are born, we breathe with a full diaphragmatic breath. Our bellies expand and contract. With age, our muscles in and around our spine and lungs stiffen, and with stress we begin to chest breath or shallow breathe. Pranayama practice teaches us to fully inhale and to completely exhale, putting equal importance on each. With full inhalation, we bring adequate oxygen to all the systems of our body, with full exhalation, we rid ourselves of the waste product carbon dioxide that is expelled through respiration. Creatures who breathe at a slower rate per minute generally have a longer life span.

The concept of pranayama is simple, yet behind it there are many complex processes at work. It is safe to say that there is an essential connection between proper breathing and health and vitality.

When beginning a yoga practice or teaching yoga, it is always best to stick to the basic practice of pranayama. There are many types of breathing exercises if one chooses to go deeper into the study of pranayama. These are the most common.

1. **Basic Belly Breathing** or **Two-Part Breath** — Sitting or lying on your back, put one hand on your belly and one hand on your solar plexus. As you inhale feel the rise of the belly and solar plexus, as you exhale feel the fall. Inhale / expand, exhale / contract. You can add to this a brief pause after each inhale and exhale.

   Teaching Tip:
   Belly Breathing Cue
   "Feel the back expand and contract. Inhale and expand the torso. Exhale and feel the shoulders move away from the ears."

2. **Durga** or **Three-Part Breath** — Always give students permission to stick with the easier belly breath if that is more comfortable. Breathing in, fill the body with the breath. Breathe in until you cannot breathe in anymore, then hold or pause for a few moments (what feels right), then fully exhale until you cannot exhale anymore air from the lungs.

   Teaching Tip:
   Durga Cue
   With new students I often count by saying, *"Breathe in for the count of three (very slow count), hold to the count of four and exhale to the count of five."* Another option is to say, *"Inhale fully, pause, and hold, then continue to fill the lungs all the way, pause again, then hold a few moments and fully exhale while thinking of completely emptying the base of the lungs of stale air."*

3. **Ujjayi** or **Victory Breath** — This is a common audible breath used in asana classes. It is often noted by the sound, which is like ocean waves or a soft snore. The breath process is said to be meditative and to control the energy in the body with one's practice. The sound allows and encourages the student to focus on the breath. This type of breathing does not often come easily and should not be forced. Students should feel free to return to belly breathing if the breath becomes labored or uncomfortable.

   Teaching Tip:
   Ujjayi Cue
   Instruct by saying, *"Sit tall and close your eyes. Breathe in through your nose and as you exhale through your mouth say 'ah' or 'ha.'"* The teacher can count *"Inhale 1, 2, 3, 4. Exhale 'ha' 2, 3, 4."* Then instruct the students to close their mouths and exhale through their noses.

This will cause a vibration in the back of the throat in the area of the glottis, the area that closes off when we swallow so we don't choke on food. So *"Inhale 1, 2, 3, 4. Exhale through the nose with the sound of 'ah' or 'ha' through the nose, 2, 3, and 4."*

4. **Nadi Shodhana** or **Alternate Nostril Breathing** — This practice balances the left and right hemispheres of the brain, helping to even out the dominance of one side of the body. We tend to alternate dominance of the brain throughout the day and that can be felt by which nostril feels the most open. This practice can be very helpful for concentration and focus before a test or speech or any activity that takes concentration and focus.

Teaching Tip:
Nadi Shodhana Cue
"To practice nadi shodhana, sit and close your eyes, taking a few moments to feel the breath enter and leave the body. Does one nostril feel more open than the other? Notice which one. There are a variety of ways to hold your fingers, but there is one that works best for me. Take the right hand and hold the thumb on the right nostril and the ring finger above the left nostril. The middle two fingers can hover over the third eye (or between the eye brows). Inhale through the open nostril (left) and then close it off with the ring and pinkie fingers. Then exhale through the opposite nostril as you release that finger (the right). Then inhale through that open side of the nose (your right) and exhale through the left." Repeat this sequence six to ten times.

Caution:
Students should also take precautions if they are pregnant, have COPD, or asthma. Always take note if someone is prone to dizziness. If they have high or low blood pressure, make sure they are not hyperventilating. If the practice makes the student anxious, have them stick with the types of breath work that are most comfortable for them. The safest method of pranayama for a high-risk student or group of high-risk students is diaphragmatic breathing sometimes called two-part breath or basic belly breathing. Encourage them before starting that if any discomfort occurs, they should stop the practice and rest in a safe place.

Asana

Asana refers to both the place and position of the practitioner, the yogi or yogini's pose or posture. Asana's literal translation is to take an easy, comfortable seat. The oldest known pose documented in writing is easy pose or sukhasana.

To recap from "Structuring a Class," there are some elements to hatha yoga that provide overall balance for the class.

1. Make sure the spine is being moved in all six directions during the class. This ensures physical and energetic balance in the body. Add safe inversions where appropriate for you or your students.

Caution:
If a student is pregnant, or has glaucoma, high blood pressure, or retinopathy, avoid deep inversions where the head is below the heart. In some cases, down dog is appropriate for pregnant women in the first two trimesters if they have no health problems and are cleared to practice by their doctor. In the case of glaucoma and uncontrolled high blood pressure or other diseases that would be contraindicated by too much blood volume to the head area, be smart and conservative and modify. Always ask the student if they have permission from their doctor to practice and have them sign a waiver. All modifications should be discussed and shown *before* each pose is attempted so the student knows how to return to the safe position at any time.

2. The class should have a beginning, middle, and an end, following a bell curve method. There should be a warm up to prepare the body, a middle that focuses on the style and type of class being practiced or taught, and a cool down with shavasana and meditation.

Next are some important notes on asanas, followed by a list of asanas that are commonly practiced. I recommend Sarah Herrington's *Yoga (Idiot's Guides)* and Diane M. Ambrosini's *Instructing Hatha Yoga* for more detail on asanas.

Asana Modifications

After many years of practice and teaching people with a variety of physical challenges, I began to develop many pose modifications. Some I learned from other teachers and some I developed out of my own experience as a student, teacher, former dance student, mother of a child who had to take years of occupational therapy, and working in the world of physical therapy.

For years, I have been teaching in what I've dubbed the "Level 1, 2, 3" fashion. Level 1 is the easiest and most modified version of a pose, with Levels 2 and 3 advancing into more difficult versions. Sometimes there are two versions and sometimes there are as many as four or five. When I become concerned that there is not a good modification for as student due to injury or other challenges, then I will offer another optional pose, which I will demonstrate.

One of my teachers, Larry Payne, PhD, is one of the founders of IAYT and a leader in the field of yoga therapy. In his trainings and his book *Yoga for Dummies*, he offers a concept that he refers to as "forgiving limbs," meaning that the student bends knees and elbow to make postures more accessible. Props are not encouraged as much as modifying the body to accommodate the posture then adding props as needed. In therapeutic yoga applications, we want to keep the student safe, so alignment for safety is important; however, the overall theme is "function over form."

Teaching Tip:
Flip It
If you are having a hard time figuring out a modification, carefully consider the purpose of a posture. Then it's often easier to think about another appropriate posture that may be a more accommodating route to achieve the same purpose. For instance, child's pose can be substituted by lying on the back in knees to chest pose. Same posture, simply turned on the back.

Personal Story:
Students as Trees.
Before the use of yoga therapy was popular or classified as a certification, I was teaching a class simply named "therapeutic yoga." It was a chair yoga class developed from my years of working with students with a variety of challenges. The class description read: "*Students with a range of physical abilities will feel comfortable in this class. Chairs and other props are used for balance and safety. Many modifications are given to assist anyone in being able to practice yoga safely.*" Earlier in this book I spoke of the "God voice." One day, I looked out on my students of many ages and abilities, from the thirty-year-old physician who was recovering from back surgery to the seventy-year-old woman who needed a walker to the young man in his mid-thirties who had cerebral palsy. Suddenly, an image of a tree appeared in my mind. Then, the trees multiplied and I saw my students as trees with a variety of limbs. With this visualization, I understood something profound. The physical part of yoga is primarily led from the spine, or trunk. The limbs can assist the pose; however, if a limb is injured or the person has an amputation, then the pose can be modified. The trunk or the spine can still move and sway in all six directions even if only a little bit, or with limited mobility. The limbs are optional! Even if the spine is limited, the brain is so powerful that the benefits of imagining the poses still have an internal effect on the body. Fascinating. Yoga is truly for everyone.

Props

Props can be used to modify poses, lengthen the arms and legs, make postures more comfortable, or deepen a pose. There are many types of props. I was taught yoga without the use of props. In fact, for the first thirteen years of my practice I never saw a prop. Years later, after I became a teacher, I attended a four-day training in restorative yoga with Judith Lasiter. In restorative yoga, props are utilized to hold poses and support the body. It is quite luxurious. Personally, I now use them as accessories in my daily personal practice. Two of my teachers in the school use props more than I do because of their background and personal training outside of my school. Stacey Reynolds studied with a teacher who was heavily influenced by Mr. Iyengar (prior to her training with me), so she uses props in most of her classes. Rena Wren went on to study with Yin Master Bernie Clark and became certified in yin yoga in which props are used to make postures more accessible. Understanding prop use can be very important depending on the style of yoga you choose to teach.

In the poses outlined below, I have recommended props you might use to help students access or deepen each pose. For more information on props I would highly suggest seeking out a teacher who has experience in Iyengar, yin, restorative, or other types of yoga that are heavily influenced by the use of props.

The Poses

In this section, I have outlined many of the most common poses in yoga. People are more apt to injure themselves in advanced postures and I recommend you train with a teacher who has many years' experience and who is very safety-oriented before teaching advanced poses. Teachers should have extensive knowledge of props, modifications, and contraindications before teaching advanced postures.

Once a student knows the basic postures, it is easy to learn how to take common poses and advance them. Learning the basics is essential to learning and teaching advanced or therapeutic applications of asana. Just like a house has a foundation, basic poses are not only preparatory for advanced asana practice, but are also the foundation of advanced poses.

Gaze or Drishti

Our gaze (drishti, or focal point), is an important part of asana. It helps us by balancing our hearing, our vision, and our sense of touch, keeping us physically stable. The direction and state of our gaze not only assists in our physical balance, but mental balance as well, helping us to concentrate and focus the mind. In standing positions and advanced postures, one can focus the gaze on something that is not moving like a spot on the wall or floor; this gaze helps to steady the body as well as the mind. The gaze is also used at times in seated positions for a focused yet relaxed mental state.

I often use "soft eyes" to describe the state of the gaze at certain points in the practice. For instance, in a seated position I will say, "*Allow your eyes to focus about 6 feet on out on the floor in front of you. With soft eyes, slowly raise your gaze as you lift your hands over your head.*" Also of note, it can be very jarring and startling to go from closed eyes to wide-open eyes without acclimating. For example, following shavasana into easy seated pose, it can be awkward to suddenly open one's eyes. So, as I'm bringing the class out of closed eyes I generally have them look down to gently open their eyes before they bring their gaze back up.

In time, internal states are heightened and balanced with practice. Closing the eyes when possible allows awareness to turn in to the more subtle effects of the practice. Throughout this section, I will note when the gaze or drishti should be closely considered as part of the pose.

Caution:

Before instructing the more advanced or more challenging versions of an asana make sure the students are truly able to do these poses correctly and are not tied up in their egos or in a competitive frame of mind. Safety should remain of premier importance. In our competitive world, people will push themselves to avoid embarrassment. As a leader, it is often our job to guide them to "take care." If the student is safe don't stress about "perfection" in this pose or any other pose.

Caution:

Headstands, handstands, and many of the more challenging inversions (head below the heart) are considered advanced asanas, and should only be done by experienced students guided by experienced teachers. As a teacher, I do not recommend teaching headstands or handstands in beginner or intermediate classes. Headstands in my lineage are usually supported by the forearms and no weight is on the head, however there is always a risk of landing on the head if one should fall. I always recommend being near a wall for support and safety. There are many inversions available that are safer for those classes. I would also personally recommend a block, blanket, or bolster under the nose in crow posture to prevent broken noses from falls.

For the purposes of this book, I have included a series of some of the most common poses. You can take the principals I have laid out below and find the information on any pose you choose by researching the many yoga books available or reading online. *Yoga Journal* is a great monthly resource.

Half Sun Salutation

Hands To Heart	Hands Above Heart Extended Mountain (Inhale)	Forward Fold (Exhale)	Half Forward Fold (Inhale)	Forward Fold (Exhale)	Hands Over Head (Inhale)	Hands To Heart (Exhale)

Full Sun Salutation

Mountain	Hands To Heart	Upward Salute (Inhale)	Forward Fold (Exhale)	Low Lunge Right Leg Back (Inhale)	Plank (Hold/Pause)	8 Point (Exhale)

Low Cobra (Inhale)	Downward Facing Dog (Exhale)	Low Lunge Right Leg Forward (Inhale)	Forward Fold (Exhale)	Upward Salute (Inhale)	Hands To Heart (Exhale)

The Poses:

1. Easy Seated Pose — Sukhasana

2. Staff — Dandasana

3. Cobbler — Baddha Konasana

4. Lateral Side Leans — Ardha Parighasana

5. Seated Spinal Twist — Paravritta Sukhasana

6. Cat–Cow — Durga–Go

7. Child's Pose — Balasana

8. Down Dog — Adho Mukha Svanasana

9. Standing Forward Fold — Uttanasana

10. Mountain — Tadasana

11. Warrior 1 — Vira 1

12. Warrior 2 — Vira 2

13. Triangle — Trikonasana

14. Pyramid — Parsvottanasana

15. Wide-Legged Forward Fold — Prasarita Padottanasana

16. Chair — Utkatasana

17. Tree — Vrkshasana

18. Locust — Shalabhasana

19. Cobra and Sphinx — Bhujangasana

20. Seated Forward Bend and Half Seated Forward Bend — Paschimottanasana

21. Shoulder Stand and Half Shoulder Stand — Sarvangasana and Viparita Karani

22. Bridge — Setu Bandhasana

23. Reclined Spinal Twist Series — Jathara Parivartanasana

24. Knees to Chest — Apanasana

25. Corpse — Shavasana

Use the references below to help you fill out the pose information in *The Mud & The Lotus: A Workbook for Students of Yoga.*

English —English language version of the posture. It's common for there to be several.

Sanskrit — Sanskrit language version of the posture. Also common to have several due to different lineages.

Benefits — Benefits for physical health and overall wellbeing.

Chakras — What chakra is balanced in the pose. You can look at the chart on page 45 "Correlating Chakras, Koshas, and the Endocrine system."

Lines of Energy — The physics of the pose—Where is the push; where is the pull. Or one might ask, What is pressing down and what is extending out? Where is the compression and extension? There are always opposing forces in the postures, which move from center. This understanding allows teachers to learn where to place their hands in adjustments and from where they should cue.

Stick Figures — Helpful in assisting with class planning and understanding sequencing; however, care must be taken not to inflexibly conduct the class according to plan. One must be prepared to adjust the class based on the concerns of those attending.

1. Easy Seated Pose

Sanskrit: Sukhasana (suka = happy, easy, and comfortable, asana = pose).

Type of Pose: Seated.

Benefits: Grounding, opens hips, balancing through entire body, assists elimination.

Chakras: All 7; Primary 1, 2, and 6.

Verbal Cues: Sit on your bottom, cross your legs one ankle in front of the other or crossed at the shins, whatever is most comfortable. Reach back and adjust your seat so your sit bones connect to the floor. Align your torso over your hips, your head over your torso. Broaden your collarbones and relax your shoulders back and down while maintaining alignment in the spine. Lift through the crown of the head. The elbows are in alignment under the shoulders and the hands will likely fall right above the knees on the thighs. Hands can be turned up for receiving position or down for grounding. You may want to imagine a string pulling through the top of your head as your sit bones root into the earth.

Lines of Energy: From the waist down to the tailbone, up to the crown of the head.

Modifications and Suggested Props: Sit on a blanket, bolster, and use blocks or blankets under the knees to ease any discomfort. To increase the opening in the thighs you can use a light bit of weight such as sand bags, but be very careful in doing so.

Assists or Adjustments: Go behind the students and gently put your lower leg to the spine, turn yourself slightly to the side, avoid pushing your knee into the back, then place your hands gently on the shoulders and instruct the student to inhale and guide your hands slightly up and on the exhale gently guide the collarbones open aligning the torso over the hips and the shoulders slightly back and down. If the student is already aligned well then skip this step, this is best for students who slump forward. If students press the chest too far forward, ask them to close their eyes and feel their body in space and see if they feel they are too far forward or back.

Variations: Easy pose is the most common pose in general hatha yoga classes and is the most available to most students. Some students struggle with this pose and will need props or options. One option is to let them sit with one leg out and one knee bent in on the opposite leg, in a half easy seated pose. The other is to allow them to sit tall with the legs out and open. The spine is most important. Remember, the legs are secondary if the student has limitations. Advanced practitioners may choose half or full lotus positions.

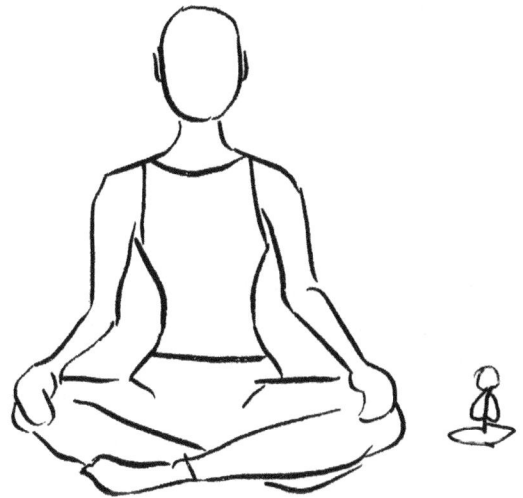

Caution *Contraindications*:
Knees, hips, and ankles.

2. Staff

Sanskrit: Dandasana (danda = stick or staff, asana = pose).

Type of Pose: Seated (can be strong).

Benefits: Mental clarity, strengthens concentration as well as increases energy in the body. Strong pose for your abdomen, pelvic region, hips, and spine. Brings alignment and stabilizes the shoulders, hips, pelvis and spine.

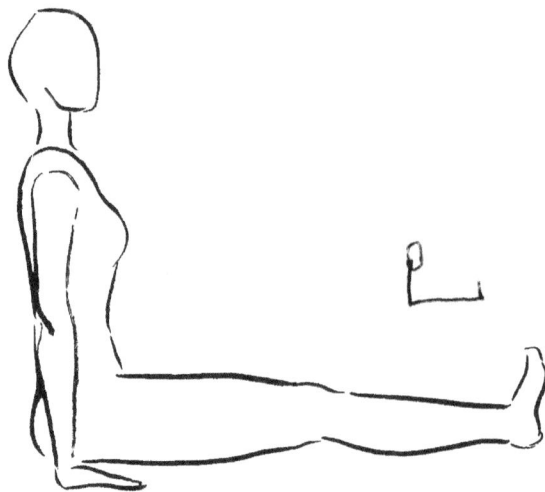

Chakras: 1–3.

Verbal Cues: Sit on your bottom and bring your seat back so your sit bones connect to the floor. From your waist or seat extend through your flexed feet, knees slightly soft. From the seat to the crown of the head lift as being pulled by a string.

Lines of Energy: Cross section at belly to head and from hips to feet.

Modifications and Suggested Props: Sit with knees slightly bent. Practice on your back. Sit on a cushion or folded blanket with the hands by the sides or up over the head or on blocks.

Assists or Adjustments: From behind the student use your leg gently as a guide without pressing into the back to support the student, gently placing hands on shoulders to lift and lengthen spine. You may also need to roll the shoulders back and down while opening the collarbones. Simply holding the hand over the top of the head can guide a slumping student to lift up to your hand.

Variations: On the back, in a chair using one leg at a time, on a cushion, on a blanket, or with hands up or down. You can bend the knees and relax the feet if the student's lower body is tight.

Caution Contraindications:
Tight hips, low back pain, or tight hamstrings.

3. Cobbler

Sanskrit: Baddha Konasana
(baddha =bound, kona= angle, asana = pose).

Type of Pose: Seated.

Benefits: Opens hips, aids digestion, and prepares women for child birth.

Chakras: 1 and 2.

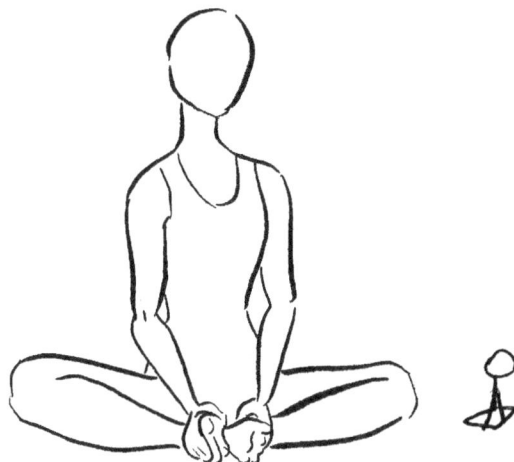

Verbal Cues: Seated on the floor, lift the fleshy part of bottom back so you are on your sit bones. Place the soles of your feet together so your legs are in the shape of a diamond. Raise your arms above your head on a big inhale and extend your spine up, then fold forward at the hips and place your hands right above your ankles (or you may hold your feet with your soles open to the sky). As you inhale bring your breath into your back extending through the crown of your head, and as you exhale relax gently forward softening the front body. Go as far as you can comfortably with your back long and extended. Avoid rounding the back until you have gone the full range of motion for your hips then you may relax the neck and head and release the hands to a comfortable place, perhaps on the floor in front of you.

Lines of Energy: From the middle body down through the seat and up through the crown of the head.

Modifications and Suggested Props: Place feet farther away from the body. Use bolsters, blocks, or blankets to adjust the seat or knees up. It may be helpful also to sit on a blanket.

Assists or Adjustments: Run your hand gently (not pressing only guiding) down the student's spine to help them relax. If the student is too far forward, instruct them to breathe and lift into your hand that is placed on the upper back. To take them deeper, you may place your hands on the crease of the hips and gently place your thumbs on the sacrum to the sides of the spine and guide the student's sacrum gently forward (always use caution). For advanced students, you may externally rotate the thighs by placing your hands on the upper thighs and rolling the quadriceps open and down with your hands.

Variations: (1) Keep forearms in on thighs and place hands up. Keep forearms on thighs and lean only as far in as comfortable. (2) Go to back and place soles of the feet together for a reclined version.

In the reclined version, you may place bolsters under the back or under the calves and feet. In some cases, such as hip replacements, the student may need to open the legs and simply put the hands on the ground.

Caution Contraindications:
Low back pain, knees, hips, groin, hernias in the groin or torso.

4. Lateral Side Lean

Sanskrit: Ardha Parighasana
(ardha = half, parigha = gate, asana = pose).

Type of Pose: Seated or Standing.

Benefits: Creates space in the lungs and heart. Massages the lungs, heart, and rib cage. Stretches the intercostal muscles and keeps the rib cage area flexible. Lengthens the spine and improves mobility. Improves circulation to the spine, heart, liver, pancreas, and spleen.

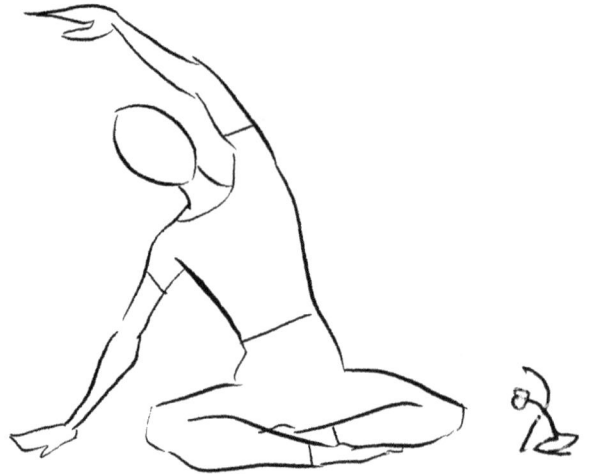

Chakras: Primary – 3; Secondary – 1, 2, and 4.

Verbal Cues: From seated, extend your arms overhead inhaling, place your right hand on the floor. On the exhale, extend your left arm over toward your right. You will be extending from the waist through the tips of the fingers while grounding the seat to the earth. Repeat on the opposite side.

Lines of Energy: From the waist to the fingers. Energy going through mid-section to the floor, and from the mid-section up to the fingers. Press down through the seat and extend up through the fingers. Watch for lazy hands or fingers—both should be active. This is a strong line from the waist to the arm to the fingers.

Notice if they are pulling out of the shoulder and encourage them to keep the shoulder head back and down.

Modifications and Suggested Props: You can use a strap between the hands, holding it taut, creating tension by pulling slightly in opposing directions. Make a C curve with the spine as you learn from side to side. This pose can be done sitting on a chair, standing, or holding on to a bar for balance.

Assists or Adjustments: If there is discomfort in the shoulder, they should soften the elbow and then the hand. Stand behind the student with one hand on the waist and guide your hand lightly in the direction of the lines of energy towards the fingers. Be mindful of respecting the student's physical space. Avoid forcing someone's arm into position; gently guide only.

Variations: Supine crescent moon (lovingly called "banana asana" in our school after a student who nicknamed it for a children's class). Lying on the floor, bend at the waist with the hands and feet moving toward the left so the body is in the shape of a banana. Repeat on opposite side.

From child's pose, walk the hands to the left and repeat on the other side.

From wide-angle forward bend or forward bend, walk the hands to the sides to make space in the rib cage. This can also be done on the floor in seated wide-legged forward fold.

This pose can be done standing, reclining, or seated in a chair.

Caution *Contraindications*:
If there are issues with the limbs or shoulders, simply move the spine in the direction of the "lean" or in "C" curve and keep arms down. Always repeat on the opposite side.

5. Seated Spinal Twist or Half Lord of the Fishes

Sanskrit: Ardha Matsyendrasana
(ardha =half, matsya = fish, endra= king, asana = pose).

Type of Pose: Seated spinal twist.

Benefits: Helps digestion, brings fresh blood and oxygen to the internal organs, massages the muscles in the back and hips, increases energy, opens the rib cage for better breathing, stimulates lymph flow, calms the nervous system.

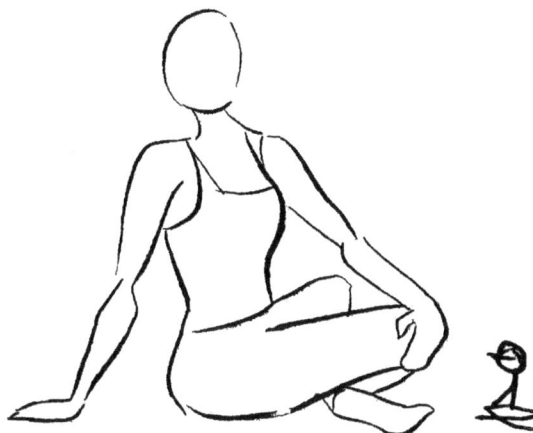

Chakras: 1–3

Verbal Cues: Sit on floor, lift buttocks back so that the sit bones connect to the floor. From easy seated pose, sukhasana, reach the arms up to lengthen the spine, then place the right arm behind you with the hand on the ground a few inches behind the spine. Take the left arm and reach across the body to the right thigh, resting the hand on the leg above the knee. With each exhale, twist deeper into the pose. Let the eyes follow the direction of the twist. Unwind from the head down as you come back to center. Repeat on the opposite side.

Lines of Energy: Up and down the spine. Inhale up through the crown of the head, exhale and elongate pressing through the sit bones.

Modifications and Suggested Props: You may prop the bottom (your seat) with a blanket. A blanket under the hand may relieve wrist pain. You may keep the legs out in front and do a seated twist with straight legs. The right arm can go to the side if a gentler twist is needed, for example if a student has osteoporosis.

Assists or Adjustments: Gently stand behind the student with your hand on the inside of the right shoulder (the direction you are turning), then place the other hand on the back of the opposite shoulder and gently guide the student in the direction of the twist.

Variations: Seated in a chair with feet on the floor. You may instruct the student to go to about

80% or less of their ability to avoid aggravating the low back, S.I. Joint (sacroiliac joint).

Caution *Contraindications*:
Hip replacements will need to do a modified version of this pose. Pregnant women should not do deep abdominal twists. Those suffering with migraines or cold symptoms should do a gentle version of a twist in place of this one. Those with low back pain should do a gentle modification as well.

6. Cat Cow Pose

Sanskrit: Durga-Go (Durga=warrior goddess who rode the back of a tiger; Go=cow, asana=pose).

Type of Pose: Forward Bend and Backbend.

Benefits: Cat Cow is a great pose for opening the spine and the belly. Massages the thymus, adrenals, thyroid, kidneys, and heart. Opens the belly and back and strengthens the core. Stabilizes the wrists, shoulders, elbows, hips, and knees. Helps with low back pain.

Chakras: Activates 1–6, Primary 1 and 6.

Verbal Cues: Come to all fours in table top (neutral spine) position. Hands should be grounded with wrists directly under shoulders, fingers spread, creating a suction-cup-type action with the middle of the hand. Press through the thumbs and fingers. On the inhale lift the chest and tailbone, hammock the middle of the back so that the chest and tailbone are lifted, and make space in the belly. Think about making space from the hip bones to the lowest rib. Feel the nice stretch in the belly. On the exhale round the back, tucking the tailbone and head. Bring the low ribs towards the hip and focus on making space in the back of the spine. Let the head relax.

Lines of Energy: In cow, the lines of energy are from the waist to the tail bone to the tops of the feet on the ground and from the waist to the top of the head, and from the wrists to the collarbones. In cat, the lines of energy are from the waist out the tailbone, and from the waist out to the top of the head.

Modifications and Suggested Props: For knees and wrists you may try folding the mat to give extra cushion. A blanket may also be comfortable under the wrists or knees. Some people like a triangle wedge for the wrists. The easiest modification for the wrists is to drop to the elbows. In instances where someone cannot be on the hands and knees (frozen shoulder or knee surgery are a couple of examples), this posture can be done seated, standing, or in a chair. For bulging disc be mindful in cat position to listen to the body—any pain is a cue to back off. Cow can be helpful for some bulging disc in the lumbar spine. Make sure students have spoken to

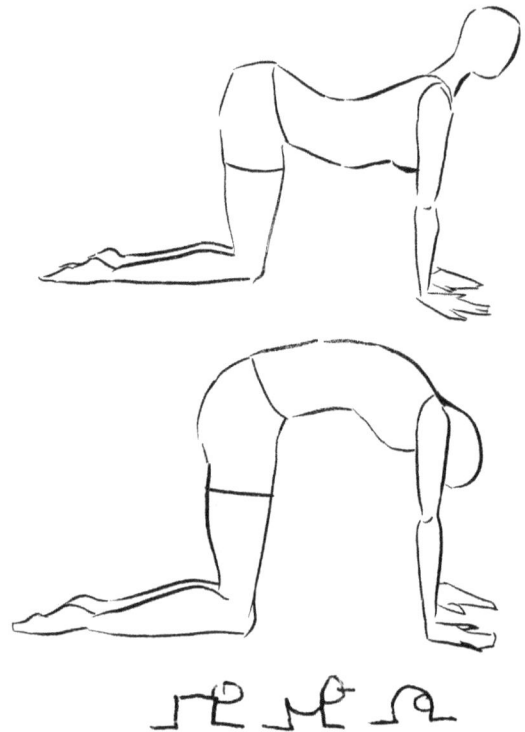

their doctors before practicing yoga. And again, be sure they sign a waiver and understand the risks.

Assists or Adjustments: Verbal cues are best here. Remind the student to keep space between the shoulders and ears. Often, I will guide with my hands as if conducting an orchestra to show the movement of the spine. Inhale and my hands go from the center up to make the shape of a bowl, exhale and my hands start up and center to make the shape of a bowl turned upside down.

Variations: (1) Invite the student to sit on the edge of a chair and do the spinal movements with the hands hovering above knees. (2) Sit on the floor and bend the knees with the feet flat in front. Hold the sides of the thighs or the shins and do the spinal movements. (3) This can also be done standing with the hands on the thighs, or holding a bar.

Caution *Contraindications*:
Wrist or knee pain, sciatica. Bulging or herniated disc (see modifications). Cat is contraindicated for some instances of bulging disc.

7. Child's Pose

Sanskrit: Balasana (bala = child, asana = pose).

Type of Pose: Forward fold, restorative.

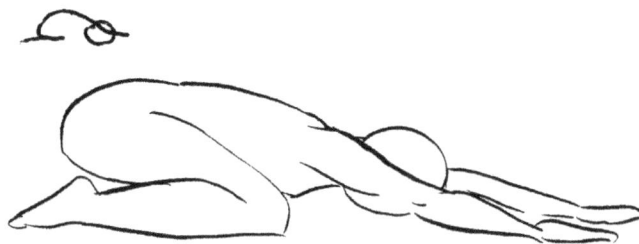

Benefits: Flexion in hips, spine, and knees. Restores energy, allows one to go inward, good for anxiety, stimulates digestion, and massages the adrenal glands.

Chakras: Relaxes 1–7

Verbal Cues: From table top, allow your hips to sink back to your heels and lower your chest as you rest your forehead on the floor. You can stretch your arms out or they may rest at your sides with hands up or down.

Lines of Energy: From the waist out the top of the head, and out the spine to the tail bone.

Modifications and Suggested Props: Place a blanket behind or under the knees. Place a block or blanket under the head. Use a bolster under the chest with the knees wide and turn the head to one side and then the other. Or simply lie on the back in apanasana (knees to chest) pose.

Assists or Adjustments: If the student's seat does not go back to the heels, that is fine. Gently run your hands down the sides of the spine, being very careful not to push down on the student's spine or back; you do not want to force the student's seat to the heels. You are only guiding the lines of energy from the waist up the spine (on the sides) to the head, and from the waist down the back towards the tailbone (low sacrum). Be very gentle, and mindful of the student's limitations.

Variations: Knees apart, feet together or apart. Arms out in front extended or soft or around the body like parentheses.

Caution *Contraindications*:
Knee pain, hip flexion, and be mindful of severe disc issues like bulging disc.

8. Downward Facing Dog or Down Dog

Sanskrit: Adho Mukha Svanasana
(adho = down, mukha = face, svana = dog,
asana = pose).

Type of Pose: Stabilization and (milder)
inversion.

Benefits: Calms the nervous system, lengthens the upper and lower body, opens the hamstrings, and creates balance in the body.

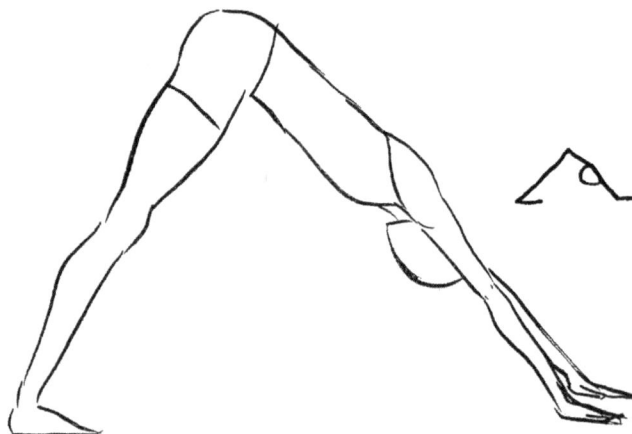

Chakras: 1–7.

Verbal Cues: From table top, lift the tailbone and knees to form an upside down "V." From the hands, extend back through the hips making a nice, long line. Keep the hands pressing into the earth with the hands grounded. The elbows should not be locked (keeping them soft but active is the safest). Keep the spine long and avoid going into a backbend or a mild forward bend. The spine stays in a nice line. Keep space in the area between the head and shoulders. Lift the heels up and, on the exhale, lengthen down through the heels. The heels will likely be off the floor a bit. If the heels touch the floor easily, create more distance between the hands and the feet. New students will tend to have a shorter distance from the feet to the hands. Leave them be at first, giving them some time to get used to this feeling. Turning upside down can be new for many adults. As time goes on, give them more feedback.

Lines of Energy: From the midline (waist). Extending from the hands to the tailbone and the hips down to the feet. Equal push and pull.

Modifications and Suggested Props: Place the heels on a rolled-up mat for support. If the student is sliding, place a hand towel under the hands. Sweat towels can be helpful here for support. Give permission language to let the students know they can go to all fours or child's pose at any point. Be patient with new students and encourage them. It takes time to work up to holding Down Dog. When we say, "rest in down dog," remember it may not be the case that this pose is "restful" for new students or students with injuries.

Assists or Adjustments: Come behind the student and place one foot on the ground between the legs slightly past the feet. Ground through your feet. Gently pull the hips slightly up and then back (hands on hip points) on the student's exhale. You may also use a strap around the thighs to gently pull the thighs back. If you need to adjust the shoulders give a verbal cue or gently guide with your fingers to move the shoulders into the socket or down and back. Pushing the ground away from them, softening the elbows and elongating the spine to the tailbone, should suffice to get the there. If they are hyperextending their backs, place your hand on the low back and ask them to move into that space.

Caution

I strongly discourage adjusting the shoulders in Down Dog. There are many risks involved so only highly trained teachers should be making this adjustment.

Variations: Especially helpful for those who need to avoid inversions or deep inversions. Hold on to a ballet barre, a counter, or place your hands on the seat of a sturdy chair (facing the chair). Extend the seat back so the body is in an upside-down L shape (if in a chair the hands will be slightly lower than the hips). The heels will be lined up slightly in front of the hips. Holding the barre or the counter, make space from the hands to the hips and lengthen from the hips to the feet. For wrist and shoulder injuries, you may also place the forearms parallel or the elbows shoulder width apart and clasp the hands. If a student is struggling with balance, consider having them try bending the knees. Placing the feet slightly farther apart than hip distance is also helpful.

For fun: Take one knee and bend it while lengthening the opposite leg slowly (avoid bouncing). This is commonly referred to as "walking the dog" or "pedaling the feet." Extend one leg at a time back and up and point, flex the foot or "floint" (point and flex combined). This posture is often referred to as "three-legged dog." If you want more, you can bend the knee bringing the heel toward the opposite buttocks and slightly opening the hip (lovingly called "fire hydrant pose").

Caution *Contraindications*:

Glaucoma, high blood pressure, retinopathy, late term pregnancy. Students with wrist or should pain can place forearms on the floor parallel (plank on elbows) or in dolphin pose with the hands locked and the elbows shoulder distance apart.

9. Standing Forward Fold

Sanskrit: Uttanasana (uttana = extension, asana = pose).

Type of Pose: Forward fold, could also be standing.

Benefits: Facilitates healthy brain function. Great for increasing energy while also promoting a relaxation response. Lengthens the spine, elongates the hamstrings.

Chakras: Balances 1–7.

Verbal Cues: Standing in mountain pose, reach your hands over your head inhaling. As you exhale, bend at the hip joint where the thighs and the hips hinge. Elongate your spine as you fold forward. Keep the knees slightly soft to protect the knees.
Hang like a rag doll breathing into the back area and with each exhale allow your body to relax and lengthen, belly toward the thighs. Keep your feet firmly planted into the ground.

Lines of Energy: From the midsection or hips down to the feet. From the hips to the top of the head.

Modifications and Suggested Props: Bend the knees as much as you need to. Come halfway up with your hands on your shins or thighs, with a straight spine. For those with hip issues or who have contraindicated conditions, try standing in front of a chair or barre, folding your arms across the seat or barre, and resting the head with the knees bent. An alternate pose would be to hold onto a chair seat or barre (or any surface), and do a modified down dog. To go deeper in the pose, pull from the calves or the backs of the heels.

Assists or Adjustments: With feet firmly planted, move the hips about an inch forward until you feel a deep stretch in the back body. Teachers should gently guide this action while standing with the feet planted and slightly open to the back of the student. Teachers may also go to the side of the student and gently guide the hand from the sacrum to the top of the spine, encouraging the student to elongate the spine. Advanced teachers may also gently touch the back of the neck at the occipital area and massage to encourage a feeling of lengthening of the muscles in the neck.

Variations: Modifications and options include:
Supported down dog
Hanging
Hands flat on floor
Palms under soles of feet
Bent knees
Holding the heels or the calves

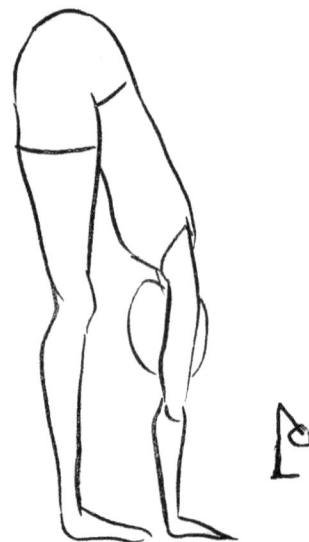

Caution *Contraindications*:
Pregnant women and those with high blood pressure or glaucoma should modify to half forward fold or use props to keep the head level with the heart rather than below the heart.

10. Mountain Pose

Sanskrit: Tadasana
(tada = mountain, asana = pose).

Type of Pose: Standing anatomical position.

Benefits: Grounding, great for ADHD, stills the mind, strong pose to strengthen and align the muscles and skeletal system. Great for the joints. Assists in proper breathing as it stretches the intercostal muscles and allows for full range of the diaphragm to open and contract. Develops awareness of consciousness.

Chakras: 1 and 6, if used for witness consciousness.

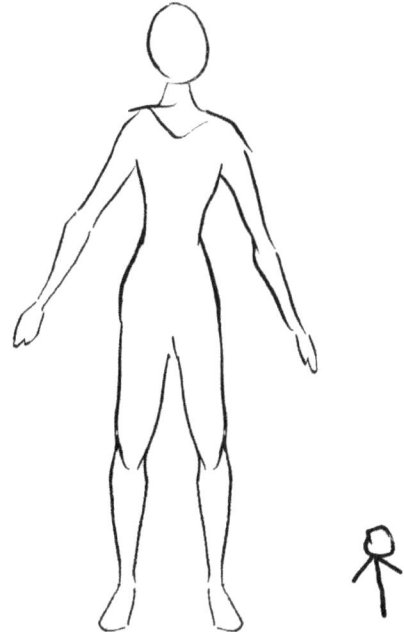

Verbal Cues: Stand tall with your feet together or hip distance apart. Ground your feet into the floor through your big toe, little toe, and back two sides of your heels. As you bring your focus up your body from your feet, begin to contract your muscles to your bones. Your thighs should hug your femur bones. Think of your pelvis like a bowl. As you breathe in, expand your belly. As you breathe out, allow your pelvis to align so that you are not tipping too far forward or too far back, as if water were in the bowl and you do not want it to spill. From the waist down, everything in the body is extending down into the earth. From the waist up, everything in the body is extending out through the head. Bring your torso over your hips, your head over your torso, your shoulders down and back, and lift your ears away from your shoulders. Turn your palms to face the front of the room and extend the joints of the fingers towards the tips of your hands. Continue to stand here, muscles engaged, space in the joints, feeling the space in the body as you extend into the ground and reach up through the top of the head, just like a solid mountain. Take three or more sets of full diaphragmatic breathing and be aware of your body and mind. When you relax, take a moment to notice the body and mind and the energy that you feel.

Lines of Energy: From the waist down through the feet, and from the waist up to the top of the head.

Modifications and Suggested Props: (1) Use a wall. Stand with the buttocks touching the wall, but do not try to force other parts of the body against the wall. (2) Use a chair or a bar to hold on to for support. (3) Have the students lie down with their backs on the floor and their feet against the wall.

Assists or Adjustments: Gently guide the shoulders down if needed by putting your hands on the shoulders and making an opening motion, guiding the shoulder blades towards one another. Hold the student's pelvis at the top of the pelvis, and guide the hips into alignment. Have the student press through the big toes to lift the arches.

Variations: (1) On the floor on the back. (2) With a chair (for holding onto the chair back). (3) Seated in a chair with feet planted, and the same actions arise from the waist up.

Caution *Contraindications*:
Dizziness or unsteadiness.

11. Warrior 1 or Vira 1

Sanskrit: Virabhadrasana 1 (Virabhadra = warrior from Indian mythology, asana = pose).

Type of Pose: Standing.

Benefits: Increases stamina, strengthens the lower extremities, stabilizes the hips and spine, great for depression, and increases feeling of strength and courage.

Chakras: Primary – 3 & 4; Secondary – 1 & 2.

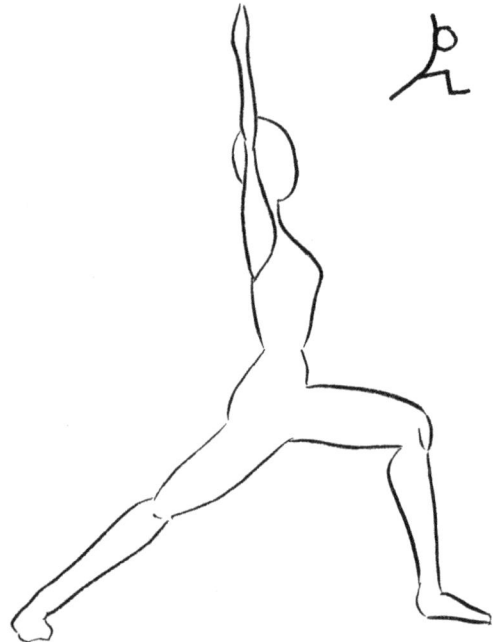

Verbal Cues: There are many ways to enter this pose. Coming from down dog is common, but not applicable for many students due to the risk of falling. This way is common in the lineage of Krishnamacharya and his son Desikachar. A safe and simple way is to stand at the back of the mat, turn one foot out slightly, and hold the hand out straight in front of the foot that is not turned out. Step out with that foot so that the foot is lined up under the hand. You will then be standing with the back foot turned slightly out and the front knee stacked atop the ankle. This version allows the feet to be more in line with the structure (distance across) of the hips so that is does not torque the sacrum. It is often taught with heel–arch alignment where the front heel is in line with the back arch, but this can aggravate the low back with repetitive practice. Put the hands on the hips and turn your torso to face the short end of the mat, and square the shoulders with the shoulders back and down. This pose is not a backbend, though that is a variation. Bring the arms up alongside the ears reaching the hands strongly to the sky. Make sure to keep the shoulders down from the ears and elongate the neck and crown of the head toward the sky. Coming out of the pose, step forward and repeat on the other side. You may also step back from the front of the mat or come up from Down Dog. There are many ways to enter this pose as well as other postures. Choices depend on where you are, what your goal is, and who you are teaching.

Lines of Energy: Waist is midline. Down through the feet. Up through the head and hands.

Modifications and Suggested Props: This pose can also be done in a chair. Imagine the pose with a chair slid under the bottom. From seated position, take the right knee out to the side, and take the back leg out behind within a range that is comfortable to the student. I tell students to imagine they are sitting in the middle of a clock with the left leg somewhere between the 9 and 11, depending on the range of motion in the hips. Turn the hips toward the bent knee, hold the back of the chair or rest the right arm on the top of the chair back. The left arm rests on the hip as you adjust the hips gently toward the knee. Arms can come up if this is available to the student. Repeat on the opposite side. Another option is to use a barre. Student holds the barre or back of chair. The right foot comes to a 90-degree angle; the back foot steps back with the foot slightly turned out. Square the hips and shoulders gently and focus the body on the lines of energy down through the feet and up through the spine and head.

Assists or Adjustments: Gently align the hips and torso holding the top of the pelvis. Not everyone can square their shoulders and hips perfectly; we do not want the students to force them square, and we do not want to attempt to adjust them square. If students' hips and torso do not move with ease, there may be other issues going on. Gently draw the shoulders down and together away from the ears, holding the shoulders and opening the collarbones. If you are comfortable with the student and believe they would be comfortable with you doing so, hold the head gently and use your fingers to place the head in alignment, thumbs at occipital bones. Be careful to not place pressure on arteries in the neck. Put your finger at the back of the bent knee. This will gently encourage the student to bend the knee and go deeper, if possible.

Variations: (1) Hands on hips, using chair or barre as listed above. (2) This can even be done in a wheelchair by utilizing the upper body and hands, focusing on the opening of the heart.

Caution *Contraindications*:
Knee issues. Keep the knee slightly behind the ankle. Press down through the feet. High blood pressure, rapid heartbeat, or risky pregnancy - keep the hands on the hips.

12. Warrior 2 or Vira 2

Sanskrit: Virabhadrasana 2 (Virabhadra = a warrior from Indian mythology, asana = pose).

Type of Pose: Standing.

Benefits: Strengthens the spine and muscles in the torso, legs, hips, and back. Good for endurance and stamina. Aligns the structure of the skeletal system and joints.

Chakras: Primary – 3 and 4; Secondary – 1 and 2.

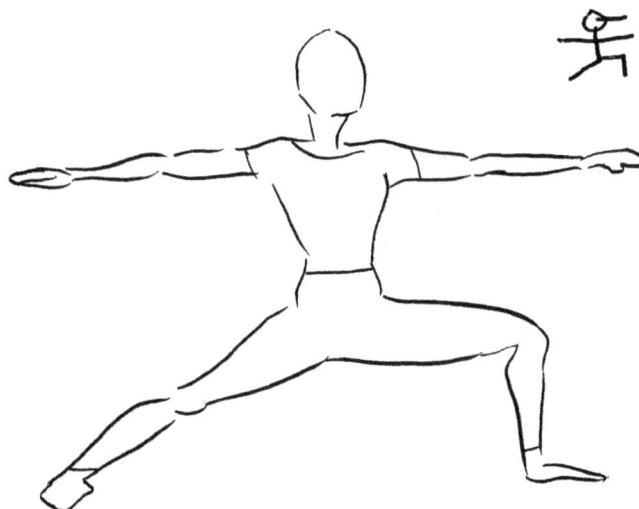

Verbal Cues: From Vira 1, take the navel toward the long end of the mat so the hip points line up with the long end of the mat or seat of the chair. The feet are pressing down into the floor with the back little toe side of the foot firmly on the mat with the feet in heel arch or heel heel alignment. The spine is now in a long line so that if you drew a line, it would would start on the floor and extend up through the midline of the pelvis, through the naval, and on through the sternum (breast bone). Then take the arms out to the sides facing the short ends of the mat from front to back. Pull the shoulder blades down from the ears, lift through the crown of the head, and gaze over the front hand which is the same as the bent knee. Repeat on other side.

Lines of Energy: Up and down the spine from the waist. Pressing through the feet and lifting toward the head. Out the arms.

Modifications and Suggested Props: Use a chair in the same way as in Vira 1. Hold onto a barre.

Assists or Adjustments: Place a finger behind the knee to encourage the student to go deeper into the pose from the waist down. Place hands on the student's torso to align the spine if the student is too far forward or back, hands on shoulders guiding shoulders away from the ears. Head should be slightly lifted. Hold the arms or hands to guide them away from each other. Verbal cues are helpful here, having the student do the "wrong" way, shifting the torso forward or back to feel what that feels like then have them do it the "right" way.

Variations: Keep hands on hips. Barre and chair as prescribed above.

Caution *Contraindications*:
Knee issues and pregnancy. Be mindful of keeping the knee behind the alignment of the ankle to not over extend. Pregnant women should proceed with caution, keeping the hands on the hips if needed after the first trimester.

13. Triangle

Sanskrit: Trikonasana
(triko = triangle, asana = pose).

Type of Pose: Standing.

Benefits: Massages the heart, lifts mood, opens rib cage for deeper breathing, stimulates elimination, and massages the hips and legs in an internal rotation.

Chakras: 1 – 5.

Verbal Cues: Stand wide on the mat with your

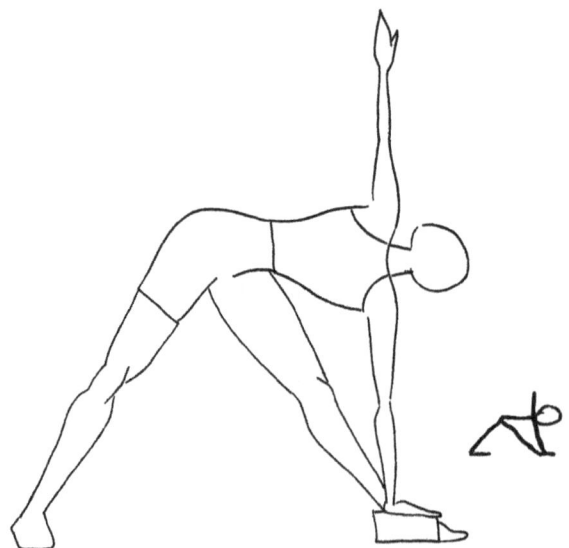

feet in heel to arch alignment (front heel lines up with back arch). Navel is facing the long side of the mat. Take your arms out wide and inhale, then exhale and lean into the front side of your foot (the foot that is facing forward and long), hips shifting forward. Place your bottom hand on the floor, along the inner shin, or on a block on the inside of your foot. Your top hand should run in line with your bottom hand in a straight line up to the sky. Open your ribs and chest while keeping your torso elongated. Your gaze (drishti) can be down or forward.

Note: Although it is somewhat common, I personally do not recommend looking up because of the lines of energy running from the midline through the top of the head. In yoga therapy and my lineage, looking up is generally done only for a moment to guide your position in space. In most medical circles, looking up is discouraged because it can lead to neck strain.

Lines of Energy: Up and down the arms, out the head, from the waist out the farthest hip and down through the feet.

Modifications and Suggested Props: Use a block or chair under the hand that would otherwise be on the floor. Stand against a wall with the back to the wall and a hand on the floor to feel the alignment of the spine.

Assists or Adjustments: Standing behind the student with your feet firmly planted, guide the upper hip in line with the bottom hip, as if the hips were stacked. Then guide the shoulders in line with one another, with the wrists in a straight line from bottom to top.

Variations: Legs wide in wide-legged forward fold with hand on the floor, doing a twist with the torso.

Caution *Contraindications*:
Those with low back pain should modify.

14. Pyramid Pose

Sanskrit: Parsvottanasana
(parsva = sideways, uttan = extended, asana = pose).

Type of Pose: Standing forward fold.

Benefits: Massages internal organs, good for menopause, stimulates thyroid and brain, good for anxiety. Assists in calming the nervous system.

Chakras: 1, 2, and 6.

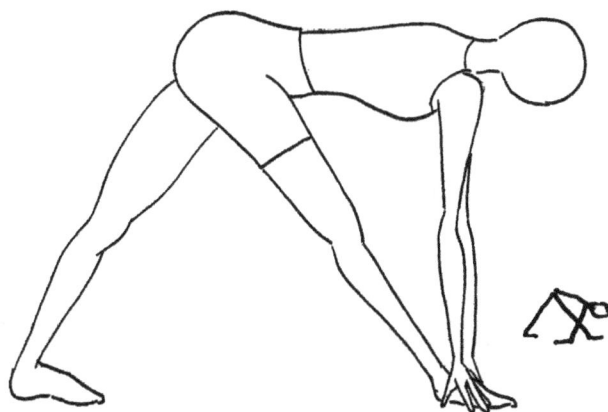

Verbal Cues: From tadasana at the back of the mat, step one foot forward. Your feet and legs will create an upside down V. Both feet should be facing forward, however the back foot may turn slightly out if that makes the hips more comfortable and level. One should try to make the hips level by adjusting the back foot. Inhale and reach your arms up to the sky, then on an exhale reach forward and down, placing the hands on the ground. Elongate the spine on an inhale. On the exhale, fold forward, walking the hands backward and the head to the knee.

Lines of Energy: Down through the feet. Down through the head. Out the back of the hips.

Modifications and Suggested Props: Use blocks under both hands as pictured in illustration. Use a chair for placing hands or forehead. Bend the front knee. If no props are available, the student can put hands on the thigh.

Assists or Adjustments: Gently pull the hip of the forward leg back while holding the opposite hip until the hips line up, but do not force this. Run your hand softly down the student's spine and massage the back of the neck to relax the head. Be mindful of personal space and boundaries.

Variations: Hold clasped hands behind the back, and open and expand the chest. Hold hands in reverse namaste mudra behind the back for an advanced version.

Caution *Contraindications*:
Anyone who should not be doing inversions. Those with high blood pressure, glaucoma, or pregnancy should all modify with a chair to keep the spine long and the head in line with or above the heart. Some hip issues may need to modify.

15. Wide-Legged Forward Fold

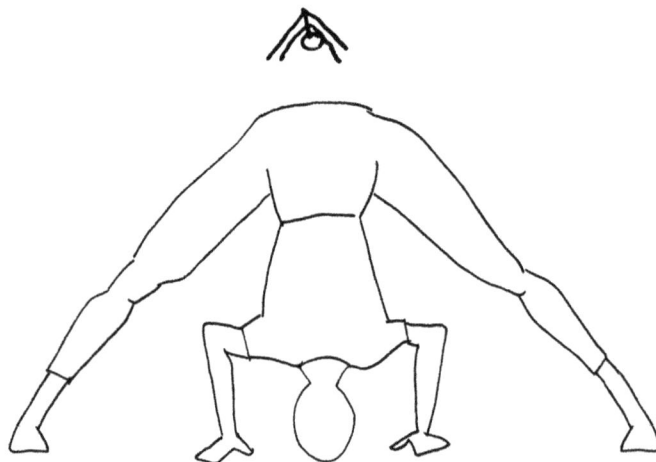

Sanskrit: Prasarita foot (prasarita = expanded, pada = foot, uttan = extended, asana = pose).

Type of Pose: Standing forward fold and inversion.

Benefits: Presses on frontal cortex of the brain, easing anxiety and depression. Brings increased blood volume to the spine and brain. Allows for elongation of the spine and torso, which can increase the ability to breathe more effectively. Good for degenerative disc disease in the spine.

Chakras: 1, 2, and 7.

Verbal Cues: Stand in tadasana facing the long end of your mat. Spread your legs wide, take your hands out wide, and line your feet up under your wrists. Inhale and reach up to the sky, expanding the chest. On the exhale bend forward at the hip joint and place the hands on the floor. The wrists will be in alignment with the shoulders. Stay here or begin to lower the crown of the head to the floor and walk the hands back with fingers facing the wall behind you.

Lines of Energy: Down through the feet. Down through the head, up the spine through the tail bone and hips.

Modifications and Suggested Props: Use a chair or block for the hands, or keep the hands on the floor under shoulders. Bend the knees. Keep a shorter stance between the feet. Put your hands on shins and hold above your ankles. Place your hands on the floor with bent elbows for comfort as you lower your head.

Assists or Adjustments: Hold the student's hips with your thumb under the hip bones and gently turn the torso down. Place your foot gently on top of the student's foot to encourage pressing through all fours. Run your hand along the student's spine in the direction of the lines of energy. Place your hands on the base of the skull and massage gently to relax the head.

Variations: Place forehead on chair with arms crossed for a little pillow. Can also grab barre or counter top.

Caution *Contraindications*:
Glaucoma, high blood pressure, pregnancy, hips and knees.

16. Chair or Powerful Pose

Sanskrit: Utkatasana (utkata = powerful, asana = pose).

Type of Pose: Standing.

Benefits: Strengthens legs, achieves mental balance and focus, tones abdomen and legs, helps achieve lasting mobility as the quadriceps muscles are vital to a long and mobile life, builds digestive heat, stabilizes joints.

Chakras: 1 – 3.

Verbal Cues: From tadasana, sit back as if you were going to sit in a chair. Focus on the seat going back. Keep the sacrum long and the abdomen toned. Raise hands toward the sky with arms aside the ears.

Lines of Energy: Down through the feet and tailbone, up and out through the top of the head.

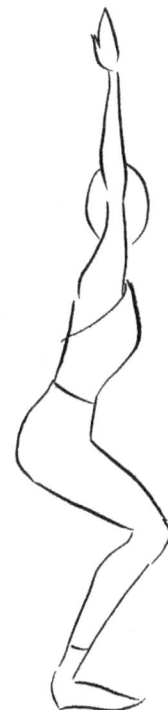

Modifications and Suggested Props: (1) Put your back against a wall and sit back. (2) Lie on the floorwith knees bent as if sitting in a chair on your back. Add a block between the knees. (3) Hold barre or chair and do a high squat without pulling on the barre or chair.

Assists or Adjustments: Gently hold the student's hips and guide hips down toward a chair pose.

Variations: Hands on hips. Keep hands in prayer, anjali mudra. Come up on toes for a more challenging version.

🤚 **Caution** *Contraindications*:
Knee pain. Those who are not physically stable or have muscle weakness. High blood pressure or high heart rate should keep the hands in prayer pose or on the hips.

17. Tree

Sanskrit: Vrksasana (vrksa = tree, asana = pose).

Type of Pose: Standing balancing.

Benefits: Strengthens and aligns the spine and legs. Stabilizes the back, hips, spine, and joints. Builds inner perceptual awareness. Allows one to build balance on the mat and in the mind and body. Strengthens the core and tones the belly.

Chakras: 1 – 3 and 6.

Verbal Cues: From standing, place your hands on your hips and shift your weight onto one foot, press through your big toe and the little toe side of the foot and through the heel (like a tripod) to lift the arch. Place the other foot at your ankle with the toes under the ankle and the heel above, at the shin below the knee, or above the knee in the inner thigh. Be careful not to place the foot on the knee, but above or below it. Elongate the spine as you inhale and raise the arms toward the sky. Keep your gaze (drishti, or focal point) fixed upon something that is not moving on the floor or the wall. Engage the thigh muscles for extra support and to make room in your joints.

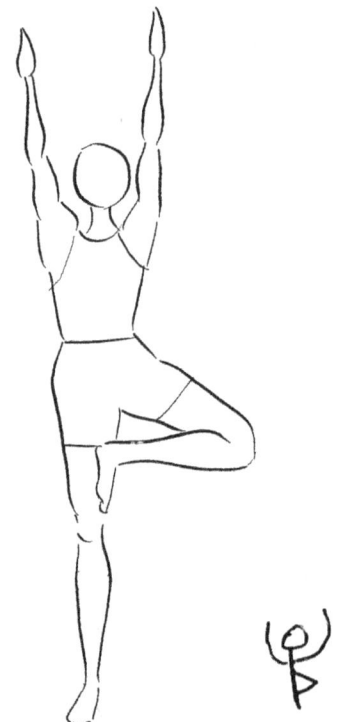

Lines of Energy: From the midline up to the sky and from the midline down through the feet.

Modifications and Suggested Props: (1) Stand against a wall. (2) Hold on to a chair, barre, or wall with one or both hands. Focus on alignment of the spine first, and add hands / arms when balanced.

Assists or Adjustments: From behind the student, plant your feet firmly and hold onto the student's ribcage on the side of the body with the foot planted. Gently take your hand on the bent knee leg at the thigh, and guide the leg back in line with the side body, only to the point that the hip points face the front. Verbal cues should be given on balancing poses before touching the student. Hands-on assists should be given after all verbal suggestions have taken place. Always proceed with caution, avoid pressing or elongating limbs and joints. It might be helpful to invite the student to practice with a wall behind them.

Variations: See props and modifications.

🤚 **Caution** *Contraindications*:
Balance issues or weakness. Hip replacements or issues with hip rotation.

18. Locust

Sanskrit: Shalabhasana (shalabha = locust or grasshopper, asana = pose).

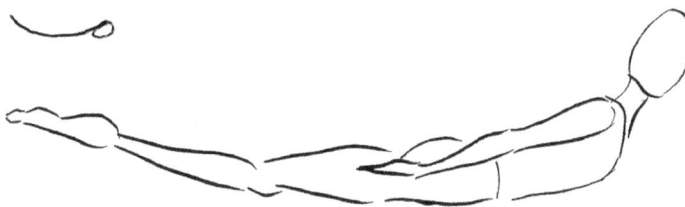

Type of Pose: Backbend.

Benefits: Good for spinal health. Especially helpful for bulging discs that bulge inward to the body, degenerative disc disease, and relief of sciatica that is caused by pinching of the nerves in the lumbar spine, but one should first consult a doctor. Massages kidneys and adrenal glands.

Chakras: Primary – 1 and 2, Secondary – 3.

Verbal Cues: Lie on the floor with the belly down. Take your legs up, keeping them extending back and out with your belly pressing down. Then lower your legs. While pressing down in your legs and belly, lift your head and upper chest. Hold for a few breaths. As you inhale, lift your legs, and your upper body and head, holding for a few breaths. Exhale, and lower.

Lines of Energy: Elongation from the midline out the feet, and from the navel to the crown of the head.

Modifications and Suggested Props: Do one leg at a time. Keep the head and arms down. Do only legs or only head and arms.

Assists or Adjustments: Remind the students to lengthen the spine and extend through the balls of the feet near the big toes.

Variations: One leg at a time, one arm at a time, using the reverse of raising one leg while raising the opposite side arm. The alternation of leg and arm offers an added cognitive benefit of strengthening and balancing the right and left hemispheres of the brain.

Caution *Contraindications*:
Pregnancy, high blood pressure, risk of stroke, heart disease. Those with low back pain should begin with half locust.

19. Cobra

Sanskrit: Bhujangasana (bhujanga = cobra, snake; asana = pose).

Type of Pose: Backbend.

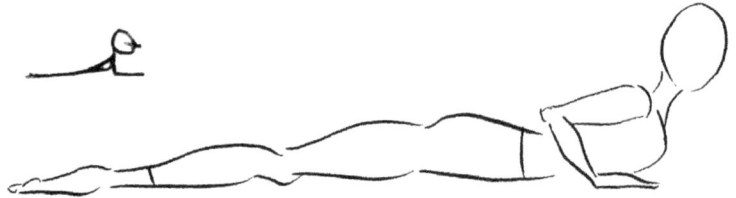

Benefits: Massages the heart. Stimulates the thymus for increased immunity. Helps relieve low back pain and sciatica. Opens the chest for good posture.

Chakras: Primary – 2 and 4, Secondary – 3.

Verbal Cues: Lie on the floor and place your hands under your shoulders with the fingers facing the short end of the mat. Allow the heels of your feet to fall open and big toes can touch or face inward. You may relax or tighten the gluteal muscles ("glutes") depending on what feels best for you. As you inhale, lengthen your spine through the crown of your head as you lift through the crown of your head, bringing your face and chest off the floor into a backbend.

Lines of Energy: From your midline up through the crown of your head and from your midline down through your feet.

Modifications and Suggested Props: Allow only the head, chin, and collarbones to lift and keep the gaze (or drishti) down to protect the neck. Many anatomy teachers in my experience have said that relaxing the glutes is easier on the lumbar spine, but others may find that it feels better to the back to flex them. Bring the hands forward and rest on forearms in sphinx pose, lifting the chest and head off the floor. Use a bolster for support under the torso and chest and push up like a low push up lifting the head and chest.

Assists or Adjustments: Come behind the student and straddle the student with your feet planted firmly. Place your hands on the student's shoulders and guide the shoulders down and back to open the chest. Only do this second adjustment if you are sure of your relationship with the student and you are aware of any health issues.

Variations: Low cobra as mentioned in the modifications, or sphinx as mentioned in modifications (see stick figure). Bring the head back into intense cobra for more of a challenge.

Caution *Contraindications*:
Pregnancy. Low back pain should begin with modifications.

20. Seated Forward Fold

Sanskrit: Paschimottanasana
(paschima = back of body, uttan=
extended, asana = pose).

Type of Pose: Seated forward fold.

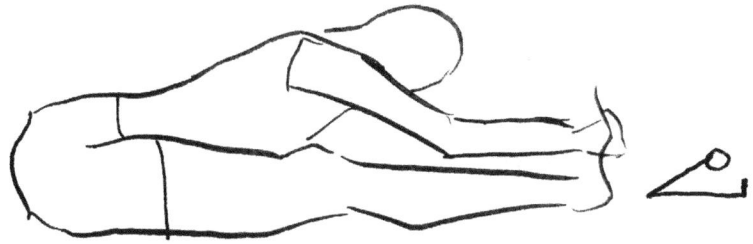

Benefits: This pose is preparatory for meditation as it puts pressure on the frontal cortex of the brain, relaxing the student. It is said that three minutes in this pose induces a parasympathic response allowing the nervous system to calm. This pose and most forward folds massage the parasympathetic nervous system inducing a calm feeling. It is used to help relieve anxiety and to improve sleep. Elongates all the muscles in the back body from the heels to the top of the head. Gives length in the spine and ribcage. Massages the abdominal organs. Beneficial to the lungs as it opens and stretches the muscles of the torso. Massages the internal organs including the abdominal and reproductive organs. Aligns the spine and extremities.

Chakras: 1 – 3.

Verbal Cues: From a seated position, take the legs out in front of you. Lift your arms overhead on a full inhale and as you exhale reach up and out then forward, placing your hands on your thighs, shins, or the outside of the feet right below the toes or on the floor. Move your belly toward your thighs. With each breath, inhale to your back and lengthen, with each exhale soften toward your legs.

Lines of Energy: From the midline out through the feet and from the midline to the crown of the head.

Modifications and Suggested Props: (1) A bolster under the chest or a block under the bolster to prop up on the far end, lying with the chest on the bolster. (2) Place a strap around the top of the feet under the toes and hold gently. Use a rolled-up mat or blanket under the knees, or bend the knees for those with tight hamstrings. (3) For those with sciatica and bulging disc, the option I give is to place the hands facing backwards while sitting up and keeping the back straight. Then, gently tilt forward at the hips keeping the spine long. There should be no rounding in the spine at all as rounding with lumbar issues like sciatica from bulging disc can increase the likelihood of inflaming the problem. (4) For those with large breasts or curves, widen the legs and place hands on the floor in the middle.

Assists or Adjustments: Encourage the students to elongate the spine from the midline to the crown of head and to flex the feet. If they are tight, have them soften the knees. Place your hands at the hip crease, your thumbs on the sacrum, and gently tilt the pelvis forward. Place your hands on the back on either side of the spine and gently run your hands up the spine toward the head. Avoid "pressing" down on the students.

Variations: See modifications for all variations.

Caution Contraindications:
Bulging disc and sciatica. Caution with pregnancy in late stages. If pregnant, should not go deep into this pose.

21. Shoulder Stand

Sanskrit: Salamba Sarvangasana (salamba = supported, sarva = all, anga = limb, asana = pose), Ardha Sarvangasna, or Viparita Karani. (All shoulder stands fall under Viparita Karani). All are versions of the pose.

Type of Pose: Inversion

Benefits: Strengthens the abdominal area, hips, and legs. Massages the thyroid and thymus. Brings increased blood flow to the face, brain, and spine. Regulates the function of the internal organs. Good pose for lymphatic drainage. Brings increased prana to the torso.

Chakras: Primary – 5 and 6 (in full shoulder stand); Secondary – 2, 4, and 5 (half shoulder stand).

Verbal Cues: For full shoulder stand (salambasana), begin lying down. Place the hands at the side body with palms down and bring the legs to 90 degrees. Engage the bandhas (locks in the pelvic floor, diaphragm and neck) and press the elbows into the earth and support the pelvis with your hands as you roll the hips up from the earth. Place the hands so that they support the hips and pelvis at the iliac crest. Bring the feet in line with the torso and make sure the elbows are not splaying out. One must lengthen and engage the bandhas to properly do this pose. Always follow up with bridge or fish posture (or their modified versions) to counter the pose. (See Section 9 for photo of modified fish pose in sample class.)

Lines of Energy: Midline up through the feet and down through the spine.

Modifications and Suggested Props: (1) Place a folded blanket under the back with the neck and head off the blanket (in reverse curvature of the cervical spine, one may be more comfortable without a blanket). (2) For half shoulder stand (ardha sarvangasana), sit next to a wall with one side of your hips touching the wall. As you come to your back, kick your legs up the wall. Place your feet flat on the wall, hands at your sides with the palms down. As you engage your bandhas, lift your hips up off the floor supporting your pelvis with your hands. For reverse process (viparita karani), from bridge pose, place a bolster under the sacrum and hips. Lower down. Place your arms at your sides with palms up. Bring your legs up. Use a wall if needed. (I was taught this method by an amazing teacher, Larry Payne, who has trained with many of the great yoga teachers in the modern world—Krishnamacharya, Desikachar, and A.G. Mohan to name only a few.) This is a great way to restore the

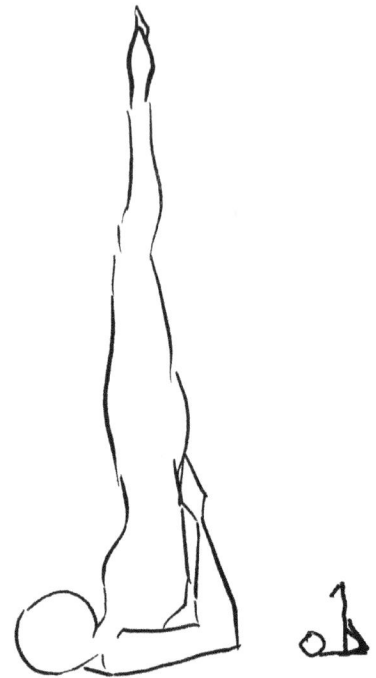

body and is safe for most people who are not contraindicated by inversions.

Assists or Adjustments: In full shoulder stand, the teacher approaches the student from the side to avoid being kicked. First, the teacher should verbally cue the student and check that the elbows are in line with the shoulders and not splaying open. The student should be fairly steady and comfortable before you adjust, and as a teacher you should be confident in your ability to do this before touching the student. From the side, gently hold the ankles between outstretched arms. On the inhale, lift toward the sky. Another method is to come behind the student (if you are certain they won't fall and kick you) and stand in a short stance warrior posture, one leg forward, knee bent, and one leg back with foot planted. Put your knee gently to the student's buttocks and hold the ankles guiding up on the inhale.

Variations: (1) Legs up the wall. (2) Using a bolster under the mid-back with the bottom off and the legs up the wall. (3) Full shoulder stand versus half shoulder stand. Advanced version is to extend the arms on the floor, placing the palms down while holding the body inverted through engaging the bandhas. (4) In cardiac rehab, we teach a simple version: Place a chair in front of you, possibly sideways may work best if the chair is armless. Place a pillow under the head and buttocks, and place the feet on the chair. (See Section 9 for photo.) Then follow with modified fish: place the pillow long with the spine and allow the head to hang off with the legs out in front or bent knees feet on the floor. (See Section 9 for photo of modified fish pose in sample class.)

Caution *Contraindications*:
Neck, wrist, or shoulder injuries. High blood pressure, pregnancy, glaucoma, hiatal hernia, or esophageal reflux.

22. Bridge

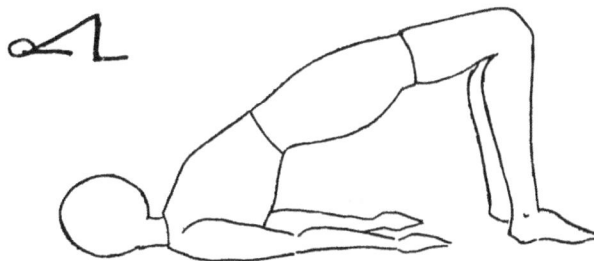

Sanskrit: Setu Bandhasana (setu = bridge, bandha = lock, asana = pose).

Type of Pose: Backbend.

Benefits: Massages the endocrine system, especially the thyroid and adrenal glands. Massages the kidneys. Tones the abdomen. Strengthens the back, buttocks, legs, and ankles. Opens the chest, solar plexus, and hips. I use this for a release of the back and follow with a reclined twist before shavasana to take any tightness out of the back.

Chakras: 3 – 5.

Verbal Cues: From your back, bend your knees so that your ankles line up under the knees. Place the palms of your hands down on the mat. On your inhale, lift your buttocks and spine off the floor. Keep your neck elongated. As you exhale, lower down slowly, vertebra by vertebra. After your last bridge (if doing several), pull your knees in to your chest to release the back.

Lines of Energy: Up from the hips. From midline into the shoulders and out from the crown of the head, and from midline to knees and down to the feet.

Modifications and Suggested Props: (1) Put a block under the sacrum on its large, flat side, or if there is more flexibility in the spine, up on its small, flat side. (2) Do pelvic tilts if the body is weak, instructing students to inhale and press tailbone into floor making space in back, and exhale and press sacrum back toward the floor while tightening the pelvic floor and abdomen. This is a good way to build the strength to eventually lift the hips off the floor. Keep feet on the floor.

Assists or Adjustments: Straddle the student and put your hands under the hips, then gently guide the hips up, opening the belly. Place your hands on the thighs and gently sweep them down toward the knees.

Variations: Take the shoulders and roll them up under you and clasp your hands.

Caution *Contraindications*:
Low back pain, knee pain.

23. Reclined Spinal Twist

Sanskrit: Jathara Parivartanasana (jathara = abdomen, parivritta = revolved, asana = pose).

Type of Pose: Twist.

Benefits: Massages internal organs. Helps slow digestion. Relieves low back pain and is beneficial for sciatica. Hydrates the discs in the spine for better spinal health. Opens the ribcage for increased respiration.

Chakras: Primary – 1–3; Secondary – 1–7.

Verbal Cues: From your back, bring your knees in toward your chest. Take your arms out to your sides in a "T" formation, palms up to roll the shoulder heads down. Inhale, and as you exhale utilize control in your low back and abdominal muscles as you take your legs to the right. Take a few breaths here. If it's available to your neck, look in the opposite direction of your knees. Inhale and use the same muscles to bring you back up, and then exhale. Repeat on the other side.

Lines of Energy: From midline out the head and from the midline down through the tailbone. Also to the bent knee from the hip area and from the rib cage toward the direction away from the bent knee.

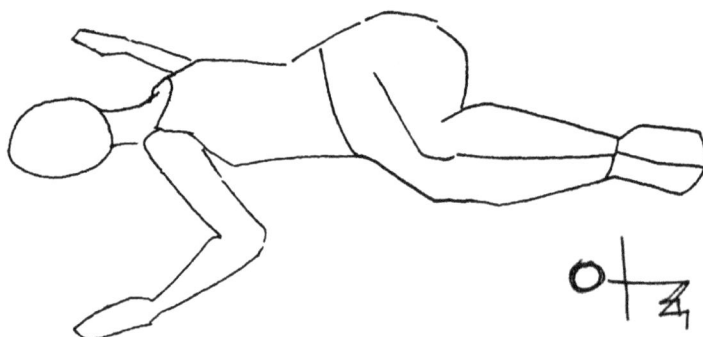

Modifications and Suggested Props: If it bothers the neck, keep the head looking up. You can also have a bolster or block under the bent knees for support. If you have any contraindicated issues, you can do this pose by allowing the legs to go over only slightly, keeping the feet on the floor and windshield wiper-ing the legs.

Assists or Adjustments: Simply put your hand on the student's thigh and gently glide your hands on the outer thigh to the knee. A deeper adjustment is to place one hand on the ribcage with the hand flat fingers facing out (make sure you kneel and are stable), placing the other hand on the thigh. As you press the thigh as stated above, gently guide the ribs away from the direction of the knee. The ribs go back and up toward the direction of the gaze (or drishti), and the thigh moves toward the knee.

Variations: (1) This option is good for those who don't need to do deep twists like pregnant women or those with the contraindications mentioned. Lie on your side with your knees bent and touching and your arms out in front of your shoulders with hands touching, similar to fetal position. Then, have someone place a bolster flat behind your back. On the inhale open the top arm and as you exhale allow it to fall back away from the direction of the knees. You may add your gaze (or drishti) as well. (2) From your back, extend your right leg out on the floor. Place the left foot on the inside of the right knee (not pressing), then hold the left thigh with your right hand, and extend the left arm into a half "T" with palm up. Then, guide the bent knee across the body with the opposite hand and gaze in the opposite direction. (This is known as a one-legged supine twist.) (3) Begin the basic pose with knees bent and to the chest, cross legs at thighs and weave legs together. Proceed to take your legs to one side on the exhale and look in the opposite direction.

Caution *Contraindications*:
Low back pain, disc injury, hiatal hernia, reflux, pregnancy.

24. Knees to Chest

Sanskrit: Apanasana (apana = downward flowing life force, asana = pose).

Type of Pose: Hip opener.

Benefits: Opens the hips and groin, releases tension in the hips and spine. Massages the abdominal and reproductive organs. Massages the lymph glands in the groin. Opens the shoulders. Helps with belly bloating and relieves gas.

Chakras: 1 and 2.

Verbal Cues: From lying on your back, bend your knees and bring one knee at a time into your chest. Hold your shins and elongate your body. Hug knees to the chest. Head can come to the knees if the student chooses to do so.

Lines of Energy: Out the tailbone and through the crown.

Modifications and Suggested Props: Bring the knees wide.

Assists or Adjustments: Place your hands on the student's shins and gently rock them side to side or gently press down and forward to stretch the back.

Variations: (1) Happy Baby—Take the legs wide, hold the outsides of the feet, and rock. Rock and roll, side to side, to massage the spine. (2) Hold the knees and make circles to massage the low back. Repeat in opposite direction. (3) Hold the shins, pulling the knees to the chest on exhale, and on the inhale allow the arms to lengthen, taking the thighs away from the belly; then exhale and pull close (the legs and the arms extend and pull back). This is a great modification for child's pose for those who struggle to get comfortable or have lumbar issues.

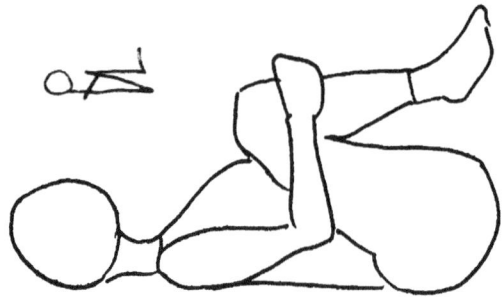

Caution
Contraindications: Pregnancy. Those who are curvy should take a wide-legged option. Those with recent back, neck, or shoulder surgery should avoid.

25. Corpse

Sanskrit: Shavasana or Savasana (sava = corpse, asana = pose). Translated to mean dead to the future and the past in this moment. Fully present.

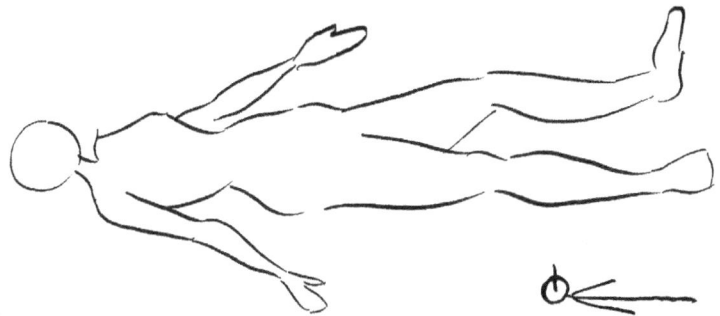

Type of Pose: Restorative.

Benefits: Calming, increases the body's parasympathetic response, calming the nervous system. Allows for openness in the body to expand the lungs and give full attention to the breath.

Chakras: 1 – 7.

Verbal Cues: Begin by lying on your back with knees bent. One leg at time, take the leg out and let the foot roll open to the side of the mat, repeat, then move to the opposite leg. Place the palms at your sides with the hands up and open (receiving position). Imagine a line coming up from between your ankles to your pubic bone, through your navel, up though your breast bone (sternum), continuing through the neck, up through the bridge of the nose, and between the eyebrows, exiting through the crown of the head. Inhale and allow your whole body to expand with breath and energy, then exhale and soften, sinking deeper into your mat.

Lines of Energy: Out the feet and up through the head from midline (navel).

Modifications and Suggested Props: Blankets can be placed under the head. Bolsters under the knees can be helpful. Cover the body with a blanket to avoid being cold. Eye pillows can assist with a deeper sense of relaxation.

Assists or Adjustments: Gently place your hands on the student's ankles as you stand with feet wide and plant your feet. Bend your knees and hold the student's legs at the ankles about a foot off the floor, then gently pull down and away from midline, and sway back and forth. After a few sways, place the legs gently back on the floor. This is a form of Thai Yoga called the reed posture, as in a reed of grass swaying from side to side. Teachers choosing to do this should be mindful of their own backs. Another option is to come to the student's head and gently place your hands on the soft area between the student's armpit and shoulder (do not get on bone or in the arm pit). Gently press back and down to open the shoulders and collarbones. Place your hands on the back of the student's neck, avoiding the arteries on the side of the neck, and gently guide your hands from the base of the neck up to the base of the spine to lengthen the neck (ears away from shoulders) as the student exhales. Gently release the head back to the floor. If you feel inclined to do so you can take your thumbs and press on the middle of the forehead (the third eye) gently, and then guide your fingers off the side and away from the student's head.

Variations: Bend the knees if there is low back pain. Go to the left side if the student is pregnant in second or third trimester. Go to belly if the student feels insecure and have them relax down with the head resting on the floor or making a pillow with the arms.

A note on bringing students out of shavasana. Have the students slowly begin to move the fingers and toes when ready to transition. Then have them stretch the arms overhead. Bend the knees, and keeping the right arm extended, have them place the left hand on the belly and roll to the right side in rescue or seed position (illustrated below). Lying on the right side has been said to give the heart a little rest. It is contraindicated for pregnancy (go to the left), and perfectly fine to give students a choice of their favorite side. Guide them through a breath or two here. Then they should use their arms to lift themselves, coming up slowly to a seated position to end class. Recall also my earlier notes about slowly shifting the gaze (or drishti).

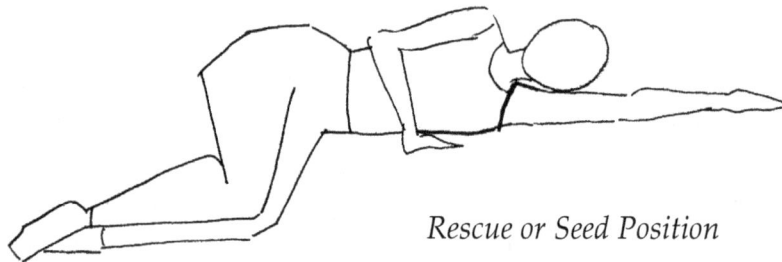

Rescue or Seed Position

Caution *Contraindications*: If someone feels insecure in this position, offer reverse corpse on the belly with the head resting to one side. A blanket can also make them feel more secure. If they have glaucoma or retinopathy, then prop the head on a blanket or pillow. People with depression or lethargy may want to sit for meditation. Pregnant women should lie on their left sides when coming out of shavasana.

Section 6: Limbs 5 through 8, Pratyahara, Dharana, Dhyana, and Samadhi

Oh, how I love limbs five through eight. They represent the ecstasy of yoga to me. You see, I came to yoga through the back door, through meditation first. I had experienced limb eight, samadhi, many times before I ever did a yoga posture knowingly. No matter how you come to yoga, it is a journey that molds you, changes you. Yoga asks us to show up, to show up for everything. To feel, to experience, to surrender. The more you let go and peel back the layers, the more you begin to know the essence of the true self and the essence of our connection to all.

At my yoga school, Balance Yoga and Wellness, I often accept people into the program who have meditation experience and little asana experience. Other students have at times made comments about this, as if it confused them as to why I would accept students who had little experience with asana practice (typically we require a minimum of one to two years of regular practice, but make a few exceptions). To me, any student who has been contemplating life is ready to take on the challenges that a yoga training can offer.

We joke about how all things in life "hit the fan" while in training. Often, I see people going through major life changes during training, some wonderful, some challenging, some both. Why is this? Life always has its ups and downs; however when we explore and discover ourselves on a deeper level, letting go of things that no longer serve us, life transition often happens. Major shifts can be challenging, but can bring a fresh awareness that often results in a new deeper contentment or happiness with life overall. The yoga journey, I believe, begins to move stuck energy and old habits in our bodies, encouraging and allowing such changes to occur. Suddenly intuition is heightened, fears and hopes are brought to the surface, and we face what is within us.

Many students expect yoga school to be eight or nine months akin to a yoga retreat, and find instead they are unexpectedly trudging through finding themselves. Much like peeling a piece of fruit to find the goodness inside, you don't get the sweetness without doing the peeling. And much like seeing a beautiful lotus absorbing the warmth of the sun at the water's surface, we have to grow through the mud to rise. When training is complete, students often remark how much they're going to miss it. The weekends we come together are full of great learning about self and others, and deep bonds are often formed. If a student chooses to surrender and be open to the process, this can be a pleasant growth experience on many levels—and indeed an experience that will continue to inform and shape them for a lifetime.

It is my belief that we are put on this earth to learn. We are faced with lessons and those lessons repeat themselves in our lives. When we learn, we do better and we live better. Or as

Maya Angelou is quoted, "I did then what I knew how to do. Now that I know better, I do better." Once we have learned one lesson, there may be more lessons of a similar but more nuanced nature. We may even feel that we are forgetting and re-learning the same lesson again and again. This is the evolution of self. It is how we grow, take shape, bend, change, and grow some more. There is no shame in our suffering, and all human beings suffer. It is what we do with that suffering that matters.

The answers of life are not outside us, they are within us. A book, a teacher, a friend, a lover, a church, or a yoga program can guide you to find the answers inside of yourself, but none of those alone can do the work for you. You must invest by doing the work—there is no way around it. You must make the journey to reach the destination, and the destination is often bound up with the journey itself. There are no easy answers. Stress is a normal part of life; becoming a yogi will not take away your stress, but it will change how you handle life's stressors.

So now to delve into the remaining limbs. Like all things in yoga, the limbs can be practiced separately or in order. My own experience leads me to "it depends" being the best "answer" much of the time. One may practice pratyahara or sense withdrawal when you need to move from external stimuli to internal noticing. Then we may or may not go on through the next few steps. It really depends on what one is practicing that day and what the intention is for the practice. These practices often are like the body, blood pumping, organs functioning, nervous system sending signals. The process can be in any given order or you may be practicing more than one limb simultaneously.

Limb 5 — Pratyahara

When I think of the practice of pratyahara, I hear birds singing in my mind. Of the eight limbs, pratyahara is one I use often on the go because I can do it easily anywhere. In many books you will find pratyahara described as "sense withdrawal." I have practiced for many years and have come to know through other teachers and my own inner guide that you will not fully experience sense withdrawal until you have sense awareness, connection, or concentration. Pratyahara to me means fully delving into life. It is being in the zone, where all things fall away except what you are focused on.

Teaching Tip:
Pratyahara Exercise
This is a pratyahara exercise I use with my students, moving slowly from one request to the next, giving plenty of time to each so that their process is not unduly cut short:

Pause after each experience and fully become aware of it before moving onto the next.

Sit with your eyes closed in a comfortable position. Let your ears focus on what you hear for a few breaths. Fully notice all the sounds around you, naming each in your mind.

Let the sense of hearing go, and begin to focus on your sense of smell. What do you smell? Fully focus on each smell around you, naming each in your mind.

Let your sense of smell go, and focus on your vision. What do you see? Name each thing you see in your mind. Even with your eyes closed, can you tell if the room is light or dark? Give yourself over to what you see through closed eyes, what you sense.

Let your vision go, and turn your attention to your mouth. What do you taste? Maybe you just brushed your teeth or had something to eat, or maybe it is a sense of nothingness. Don't judge it. Just name it in your mind and let it go.

Now turn attention to your skin. What do you feel? Your clothes against you, perhaps a breeze, the cool or warm air, your seat on the floor. Delve into it with your entire being, allowing yourself to fully feel it. Now let it go.

Limb 6 — Dharana

Limb six, dharana, is the limb of concentration and focus. Immediately, you could see that the fifth limb, pratyahara, was one of concentration and focus as well. Dharana is fully allowing your mind to be on the task at hand. It may be watching a candle flame, watching a child play, listening to music, or sitting still and feeling your breath. It is simply "noticing."

Personal Story:
Lilias Folan's Yoga and . . . ME!
One of my favorite dharana exercises was taught to me by the first person to introduce me to yoga, Lilias Folan. I was a young child of the 1970s, and watched hours and hours of PBS. Lilias's show, *Yoga and You*, aired on PBS from the 70s to the 90s. I was an only child and up for anything, so I enjoyed watching the show and doing the exercises along with Lilias. Later in my life, it became one of my goals to study with Lilias, whom *Time Magazine* has called the "Julia Child of yoga." In 2012, that goal became a reality! I spent a weekend with her in a workshop, and was able to see a concert with her and a few other yogis. I am so grateful for this experience.

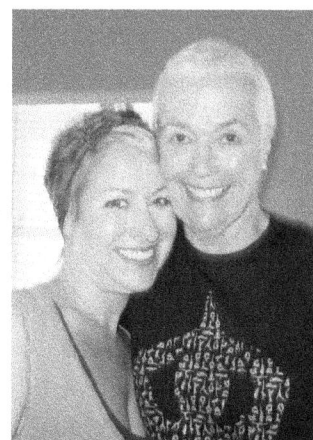

Butler & Lilias Folan, Summer 2012.

Lilias Folan taught me many things that weekend, but one of my favorites was this exercise in dharana. If this does not quite work for you, do not judge it; rather, examine the practice in your mind and know that your mind is an amazing instrument for growth. Science has shown us that our minds have more control over what happens in our body than was once thought possible.

Teaching Tips:

Sit comfortably and take your hands together in front of you. Line them up at the lines of your wrists. Now look closely and you will see one hand is slightly longer than the other. Name it in your mind. Now put your hands face up on your thighs and breathe. Focus on the shorter hand. As you breathe imagine that hand extending and getting longer. Feel the bones in the hand extend. Inhale into the base of the fingers in the first joint, exhale and imagine it lengthening until it has reached the second joint. Inhale into the second joint and exhale and imagine the fingers lengthening to the tip of the fingers. Breathe in and out and as you exhale, imagine the fingers and the hand extending and getting longer and longer. Now, open your eyes and put your hands back together and see if the shorter hand didn't even up or get longer than the previously longer hand. It is an amazing and crazy thing that for many people the initially shorter hand will be longer than the other hand after this practice.

One simple lesson of dharana practice is *"What we focus our energy on grows."* If we focus our energy on sadness, then our sense of hopelessness grows. If we focus our energy on health, wellbeing, and contentment then we will have an overall sense of wellbeing.

When you are in meditation, you may practice this by simply focusing your mind on the breath by noticing the rise and fall of the chest and belly.

Limb 7 — Dhyana

Dhyana means meditation, but if you are following the limbs in order, you may already be in a state of meditation. It is said that it takes the brain up to ten minutes to reach a point of meditation where the brain, body, and mind let go of all the chitter chatter that so often clogs up our "monkey minds." Practicing pratyahara and dharana helps to calm the surge of thoughts and feelings that run through our brains so that we can reach dhyana, a state in which love flows through us and creates a higher than usual vibrational frequency. When this stage is reached, acceptance comes that we can detach in a healthy way from our thoughts and escape the constant noise that fills our brains.

If I practice meditation, I learn that in life I can be sad and obsess about a certain issue, such as a fight with my partner. However, I know I must go to work so I can take a few breaths, allow myself to know that I am not my fight with my partner, that the situation or feeling is not me, it is just a feeling. This practice allows me to move beyond those thoughts and feelings, let go, and do my job, knowing that ultimately no matter what happens, everything will be okay. Those thoughts and feelings do not have to control me. My feelings are simply feelings; they are not necessarily facts that I have to react to. Whereas in my youth I might have been tempted to call in sick from the physical and mental pain stress caused me, my years of practice have helped me to learn healthy detachment.

Studies have shown that the brain is strengthened through meditation. The ability to control one's thoughts and actions are increased with control of the mind. A parasympathetic response happens in the nervous system when one meditates. The parasympathetic nervous system is responsible for "rest and digest" and the sympathetic nervous system controls our "fight or flight" responses. They are both a part of the autonomic nervous system which is responsible for involuntary functions of the body. Meditation allows the brain to control the flight or fight response and get the body and mind back into homeostasis or balance. This state of calmness or oneness is attained through all eight limbs, mediation being the pathway to the state of dhyana.

Personal Stories:
My Meditation Practice
After I have walked and done my asana practice, I often read a daily meditation from *Journey to the Heart* or *The Language of Letting Go*, both by Melody Beattie. Then I sit. I may contemplate what I have just read, or I may just sit and notice what comes up. If sad feelings come up, I internally become objective and say to myself, *"That's a sad feeling,"* and let it go.

To carry my meditation practice with me throughout my day, I sometimes tune in to what is called the "witness observer." This is when you pull back your mind and observe your thoughts and actions as you would if they were not your own. For instance, I may reflect on a situation where I reacted to something in a way that does not please me. Then I would say to myself, *"That was a response of fear."* I don't judge it. I don't do anything except notice it, and let it go. By doing this practice, the next time the situation comes up deep in my subconscious mind, I am aware that it was a reaction of fear and I can have more control over my actions and reactions. This method is often called the A.L.L. method: Accept, Label, and Let Go.

Meditation and Hypnosis
As a Yoga Therapist (C-IAYT), I study many facets of the human mind and how I can use different techniques with my clients. Recently I started getting curious about the similarities between hypnosis and meditation. I discovered that what I had been doing and teaching for many years was more similar to hypnosis than I knew! When a person is hypnotized, they are in such a state of relaxation that the subconscious mind is more apt to take on suggestions. The difference in meditation and hypnosis is in meditation we keep the person conscious or awake. In the subconscious mind, we do things with-

out thinking about them like the way we move, our body language, our simple actions that we may not even realize we control. Have you ever been driving down the highway thinking of something and missed your turn? You were thinking about something else, but your subconscious mind had been driving so long that it just drove on without giving the act of driving much thought. This is how we can essentially do two things at once.

What might we, as teachers and students, learn from hypnosis to inform our meditation practices and teachings?

Teaching Tip:
I use this approach with my yoga therapy clients, and adaptations of it can be useful in any type of class or for self practice. While on their backs, go through a series of exercises to relax the physical body, such as tensing and releasing the muscles progressively. Then guide students through a series of exercises that relax the mind. For example, have the student visualize a magic carpet ride where the mind sees things such as traveling to a place that is relaxing or comforting. The carpet should ultimately land in a place that is mentally and physically safe. The mind should be in a state which is suspended between sleep and awake or consciousness and unconsciousness. This is when suggestions take hold, so it is time to add affirmations or visualization. If you know the student well, or if this is for your personal practice, you can suggest visualizing what it is that the student wants in steps while taking in all the senses. *What do you see? What are you wearing? Who is there? What does it smell like?* Then you might make suggestions and have the student/client or yourself repeat them in the mind in the present tense as if they are already happening (e.g. *"I am healthy," "I am whole," "Cigarettes have no hold on me," "I am a good wife," "I am a best-selling author,"* etc. Then say to the student, *"In your daily life, allow these things to take hold in your body, mind, and cells."*) Then you will slowly bring the student back by guiding them through a series of noticing things with the body and mind. Notice your skin and how it feels and then drop into your body and feel your breath. As you breathe in you might have them say to themselves something quietly, "It is so," and as they breathe out, let it permeate their body and ask them to let go of negative thinking. Or simply ask them to take a mental snapshot of what this statement looks like to them and imagine what it looks like in real life. Have them see themselves doing the action they just imagined. After this visualization is brought to a close, ask them to stretch and come to their sides for a few breaths, then transition back and sit up with their eyes closed. Take a few moments to sit and just be. Inhale and bring arms overhead, exhale and bring hands to your heart center in Anjali mudra (hands placed together at the center of the chest, symbolizing sealing the practice).

Limb 8 — Samadhi

Samadhi is the state of oneness or bliss that one feels when one reaches a state of utter surrender and connectedness in which the ego disappears. Samadhi is a heightened state of awareness where all things fall away and there is a sense of peace and oneness. This final attainment of pure bliss may or may not ever be achieved, but is something to work toward through practicing the other seven limbs of yoga.

Often the minute one recognizes they have reached this state, the mind goes *"Oh, I am here! Eureka! I want to stay here forever!"* then the sense passes quickly. In this state, there is no feeling of hate or sadness or anything at all except pure ecstasy. One may see colors or lights in the brain and possibly feel a sense of pulsing in the body. At times truly it is simply a deep sense of relaxation and peace. At other times, it feels like what many people recount from when they've been on the brink of death or are crossing over.

Samadhi is a complex concept to put into words. If you have never acknowledged or recognized this blissful feeling and you go searching for it, you can feel exasperated and you may even struggle with shame if you perceive that you cannot find it. It only comes with complete surrender. This often happens for people in other instances where they are extremely happy or focused and they do not recognize it as a feeling of samadhi. Though you may not find this each time you practice, with time you will find bits and pieces of it scattered throughout your daily life. As stated earlier, all the limbs work together so you may feel different degrees of bliss as you begin to practice all eight limbs in your daily life. You may feel samadhi as you practice pranayama or asana. You may feel it as you meditate. You may feel it as you listen to the birds sing, make love, pet your dog, hug your child, and listen to your elders. It is always there. Practice of the eight limbs allows us the door to access it.

Meditation in Practice

Throughout this section of the book, I've given examples of meditations that I teach. There are many types of mediation practices. You can try many or just stick with one. One organization for which I'm a contractor separates out deep relaxation, meditation, visualization and so on. One easy way to look at this is to say that it is all mindfulness practice.

As you study, you may find recommendations that you should practice at certain times of the day, for certain lengths of time, sitting or lying on your back, etc. What I would say to you is find what works for you. Five minutes a day is better than none at all. If you enjoy what you are doing, you will do more of it.

For further information on meditation I recommend going to UCLA's website and typing "meditation" in the search bar. I also like the app *Insight Timer*. There is so much information on the web and in books you need not look far for guidance.

As you learn more about it, your entire life may become a meditation. You may find yourself sitting in a doctor's office quietly focusing on two hawks flying around outside the window with no other thoughts. You may find yourself sitting at the ocean with your eyes closed listening to the waves and realizing on a cellular level that the world is a big place and all living things are connected in some way. You may be sitting on your mat and focusing on your breathing or find yourself in a yoga class with a great sense of relaxation and peace. You may find that after you leave class you no longer have the anxiety and fear you came in with. This is the practice of yoga; this is meditation.

As students and teachers, do not skimp on this part of your practice. The greatest gifts of yoga are here. Allow yourself to slow down and find time to contemplate life, wherever you are, wherever you go. The mind is your greatest tool. My personal experience is that when I pray I talk to God; when I meditate I listen to God. My biggest revelations in life have come when I sit in quiet stillness.

Section 7: Yoga Business Basics

"It is business, but it's never 'just' business."
~Courtney Butler

The subject of business in yoga is so vast and broad that it is challenging to address every avenue that can be taken by a yoga teacher. I would advise finding a mentor you trust who is willing to be honest with you about what the world of yoga has been like for them. If you want to open a studio, then find a studio owner that you will not be competing with who will share with you. If you want to teach corporate yoga, do the same, and so on.

The best advice I can give is always look to the yamas and niyamas before deciding, and ask yourself if you are following the Golden Rule—doing unto others as you would have them do unto you.

Finding Work and Getting Paid

When you start out, it is best to take classes in the places you would like to work. Yoga styles vary greatly so you may find that you like one style or vibe better than another. Then ask the teacher, administrator, or owner if you could be on the sub list. They may ask you to try out. This is common as they may want to see you teach. You can also apply at various places like gyms, yoga studios, community centers, colleges and any place that has a large open space and is willing to host a yoga class.

The amount yoga teachers make varies depending on where and what they are teaching and for whom they are working. With each teaching assignment, you need to determine if you will be a contractor or an employee so you understand the laws and expectations than can or cannot be placed on you. Sometimes you have a choice and sometimes you do not. As an independent contractor, taxes are not withheld from your check; rather, you are responsible for paying taxes and you will be asked to complete a W–9 for tax purposes. If you are an employee, you will be asked to complete a W–4 and taxes will be held out of your check just as with any other regular employment. Consult an accountant and/or attorney for more details on the differences between of being classified as an employee or independent contractor.

Below are some examples of different places that might offer teaching opportunities and their possible pay scales or structures. If you are an employee, you would be well advised to ask if there is a policy about you teaching in other places. The contractor, administrator, or owner may not want to hire those who teach at competing businesses. Communication is the key to avoiding these challenges and future hurt feelings.

Gyms and Colleges

Working for a gym or college, you will usually be classified as an employee and they will withhold taxes from your paycheck. They will likely tell you what times they have available for you to teach. At the time of this book's publication, pay rates vary from $12 to $35 an hour depending on geographical location. Some may pay a certain amount per student; however, this is more common in a studio.

Studios

Studios all approach teacher payment very differently. Pay scales range from $13 a class in smaller communities to $65 a class in large metropolitan cities. There are often sliding scales.

Studio Pay Rate Examples

Base Rate + Pay Per Student
Base pay = $10. Studio pays + $4 per student after the first 5 students.

10 students come to class
5 at base pay of $10 = $10
5 additional students at $4 an hour = $20
_____
Total pay for the class = $30

Per Student Rate
Studio pays $5 per student
10 students attend class
_____
Total pay for the class = $50

Sliding Scale Rate (I used this model at my studio)
$10 for showing up
$20 for up to 4 students
$25 for up to 10 students
$30 for 11 to 15 students
$35 for more than 15 students

For Studio owners, Prospective Owners, and Teachers

Staying in Business

Being a studio owner and understanding the position of the studio owner or administrator provides valuable lessons in the yoga business. Classes barely pay the bills in many cases. Of course, it always "depends" on your unique situation, however I find this holds true in most cases. I'm a research fanatic and a numbers person. Learn from my mistakes! This is actual information from my many years as an administrator, teacher, studio owner, school owner, and private yoga therapist.

When I was an administrator of a large nonprofit, I paid using a sliding scale based on the credentials for the teachers who worked under me—the more qualified the teacher, the more the teacher was paid per class. My boss told me my teachers were going to price themselves out of a job. When we hit a budget crisis, I was instructed to only use the lower-paid teachers and give them more work because they were averaging as many students as some of the higher credentialed teachers. Long-time teachers usually have a more consistent following. Experienced teachers may have 10 students on average who are very loyal to them and have followed them for 10 years. Newer teachers will often have more sporadic class sizes as they build a clientele, perhaps 10 one week, 5 the next, and 15 the following, then 2 the next. So, I don't recommend paying on credentials; however, there are ways for more credentialed and skilled teachers to make money. Those are the teachers to whom I would give more of the private lessons and other similar opportunities.

It is also vitally important that a prospective studio owner understands how much it costs to keep a studio afloat financially. It takes approximately 75% of the total income from classes to run a studio. If you have 10 classes per week at an "average" of 10 students per class and the "average" class price is $13, you are making $130 a class or $1,300 a week for classes. If you pay your teachers ½ the price of a drop-in rate, let's say $7.50, then you will likely be short on the money to pay your rent, insurance, taxes, supplies, advertising, etc. **I do not recommend choosing an arbitrary amount to pay your teachers if you want to stay in business.** I recommend you pay 25% of the "average" class total income.

Every class should be on a 3–month trial basis. It the class does not make the minimum, it needs to be moved, removed, or have a change in teacher.

If your drop-in rate is $15 and your best package price calculates to $10 per class, your average price per class is somewhere around $12.50. You do not want to pay more than $3.13 (25% of $12.50) per person or you will be in the hole. This may sound jaw-dropping to a teacher, but this is the reality. The owner needs to be paid, plus there are enormous expenses to keep a brick and mortar business afloat. Using this example, I would not allow my pay for teachers to run over $31.30 on average for a class. This is how I came up with the scale I used. In a metropolitan area where class sizes are bigger and the cost is more you can adjust these numbers and pay your teachers more, however you must remember that rent and other costs may also be higher in those areas.

Example: Small Town Yoga Studio

Stats for an average small town studio:

- Average class size= 8
- 10 classes offered per week.
- Town's average salary is only $35,000 per household (information from USA.com or Trulia.com)
- Packages run $80 for ten classes, or $8 per class.
- Drop in cost is $10
- ½ the students are on package and ½ are drop in.

  □ Take the number of total students in one week and divide by 10 to get your average class size.
  □ In a given week, 80 people sign in. 10 classes per week are offered. Divide 80 by 10 and come up with average class size as 8.
  □ Assuming 80 customers per week, half paying $8 (40 x $8 =$320) and half paying $10 (40 x 10 $400), then the studio is making making $720 per week ($320 + $400).

Small Town Yoga Studio Fixed Rate

  □ If the studio pays teachers $5 per student ($5 x 80 = $400), then only $320 will remain to pay the owner's salary and bills for the entire week. Not a good idea!

Small Town Yoga Studio Sliding Scale

Let's look at the pay scale I used at my studio. I am in a medium-size tourist town and the average class size is about 8.

The average teacher would make $25 a class on this scale:
$10 for showing up
$20 for up to 4 students
$25 for up to 10 students
$30 for 11–15 students
$35 for more than 15 students.

On this sliding scale, Small Town Yoga is bringing in $720 a week and paying teachers on average $250 a week (10 classes of 8 students at $25 per class). This leaves $470 to pay the bills and the owner's salary.

Small Town Yoga Studio Monthly Expenses

Total Income = $3,096/month ($720/week x 4.3 weeks (31 days/mo))

Rent $500
Insurance $100

Owner's Administrative Fee $800
Contractors $1,000
Taxes $300
Supplies and Cleaning $100
Advertising $150
Accountant $50
Miscellaneous $96

_____

Total Expenses = $3,096/month

You can see very quickly that the greatest monthly expense is teacher compensation. **Therefore, many owners will need to teach most of the classes. This owner would not be able to survive without another source of income.**

Example: Urban Yoga Studio

Stats for an average urban studio:

- Average class size is 15 students
- 28 classes per week
- Average income per student is $60,000
- Drop in is $20
- Class packages are 10 classes for $140 ($14 per class)
- Half are drop-ins and half are on packages, for an average price per student of $17

  □ Take the number of weekly students on average and multiply that times the average price per student. 28 classes per week x 15 students per class = 420 students per week. 420 x $17 per student and get on average $7,140 per week of income.
  □ Multiply that times 4.3 (31 days/month) and monthly income is $30,702. (Before you decide to move to the city remember you must consider the cost of living and that many things cost more. Small towns should not try to compete with urban cities on charging and pay scales.)

Urban Yoga Studio Sliding Scale
Let's use my pay scale above, but make a few changes.

$25 for showing up
$35 for up to 4 students
$50 for up to 10 students
$60 for up to 15 students
$70 for more than 15 students

The average pay to teachers is $60 so the amount set aside to pay teachers is $1,680 based on 28 classes per month.

Urban Yoga Studio Monthly Expenses

Total Income = $30,702/ month ($7,140/week x 4.3 weeks (31 days/mo))

Rent $7,500
Insurance $500
Owners Administrative Fee $4,000
Administrative Assistants $2,000
Teacher Pay $7,224
Taxes $3,700
Cleaning $600
Props and Other Supplies $800
Advertising $1,800
Accountant $250
Miscellaneous: money held back to pay for big expenses like renovations, replacement cost of props and preparing for a retreat, or putting money down to host a large workshop $2,328.

Total Expenses = $30,702/month

As you can see as a teacher and a prospective business owner, there are many expenses that come along with owning a brick and mortar business. Taxes alone range from 10 to 15% every month!

A word about retail. I did not include the cost, profit, and loss of having retail. That is another conversation. There are a ton of expenses and headaches with retail. It would be advised that you feel comfortable in that area or at the very least start slow and learn because it can end up being a huge expense if you have a ton of retail sitting around that you can't sell.

Determining Per Class Charge

First, look at what other businesses in your area are charging for yoga. If there is no other yoga offered, look at the cost of other extracurricular activities in your community. If dance classes cost $15 a class and karate costs $75 per month, that is a good idea of what your range is in your area.

If you are in an area with a lot of cheap yoga at gyms, then be mindful of what you are offering and how much you can charge. It was very difficult for me to compete with gyms in my area because they were in very close proximity to me and I had trained most of the teachers, so there were many registered yoga teachers. You could pay $37 per month to go to the local nonprofit and get all the yoga you wanted; however, you had to put up with loud noises and a gym atmosphere. Therefore, I offered a spa like feel and charged $10 a class. My sister studio in an urban city an hour away charges $15 per class. I highly recommend that you do your research before you go set your per class rate. It is true that you can always change it later, but your first number sets expectations that may be difficult to change.

As of the publication of this book, the average charge in Arkansas is $10 per drop in. It is $5 in some very small towns and $20 in larger metropolitan cities.

Income Sources for Yoga Teachers

For new teachers, I suggest taking whatever you can find that fits your schedule. In my experience working with teachers, it's best to spend a couple of years teaching before you embark on any expensive endeavors. Again, it always depends on many factors and your personal financial situation.

Most yoga teachers have full-time careers, or only want or need to work part time. Many yoga teachers are reliant on their current careers and complimenting them with yoga. Some examples are school teachers, medical professionals such as doctors and nurses, and social workers. Many of the people I train work in colleges and teach in higher education, or in teaching or developing programs for their communities.

Making an Income Working for a Studio

Teacher pay averages $25 per class as an average for a midsize to larger studio in Arkansas and throughout most of the South. When I travel to larger cities, I have seen pay as much as $65 a class. In smaller cities, I've seen it as low as $10.

To get started, you might teach several classes a week and promote the heck out of your classes via the marketing means mentioned in the marketing section of this book. Slowly, focus on building your clientele. To supplement, ask the owner if you can work another area of the studio like the front desk. If you have the experience and are prepared, ask if you can take private clients in the studio from among your clients. Or reach out to special population like "Yoga for Curvy Women" or "Special Needs Children" with which your skills and experience match up.

Let us look at a scenario.

You have worked for two years at ABC studio and built up to 4 classes per week averaging 15 clients per class. You are being paid $50 a class for $200 a week.

On the two days per week you teach, you work 5 hours at the desk at $12 an hour = $60 x 2 days is $120 a week.

You teach 2 private clients per week at $75 per session and you pay the studio 20% ($15) so you make $60 per session for $120 a week.

Earning $200 for classes plus $120 for front desk work and $120 for private clients is = $440 a week or $1,892 per month. Not bad for a total of about 18 hours of your time. (I included arriving early and closing with classes and private clients.)

Add an intensive once per quarter on a special topic for 15 people at $60 each = $900. Subtract 30% for the host studio (- $270) and you make another $630.

Depending on the rules in your state, you may be a contractor or an employee so you would need to check those laws. Remember if you are a contractor you need to pay your own taxes, so don't forget to subtract that percentage from your anticipated income.

Working with Other Businesses: The Percentage Approach

This is often considered the safest route if you want to branch out on your own. You might want to teach in a church, dance studio, or any place that has wide open space and an atmosphere you can use for yoga. The going rate for teaching in a space is about 20 to 30%. For hosting a workshop, it is 30 to 40%.

For example, you host a yoga class and 10 people attend (this may take time to build up) and you are charging $10 drop in. You will make $100 and pay the host $25. You have made $75, but you are responsible for things like advertising, your taxes, your props, etc.

Renting Space

Local Dance Studio Space Rental Example

You want to figure out if it's economical to rent space at a local dance studio. They charge a flat fee of $25 to use the space for two hours (this gives time for set up and clean up).

- You charge $35 per month for four classes.
- You have an average of 4 students pay up front, so you collect $140 and use most of this income to pay your rent of $100 ($25 x 4 classes).
- You average 10 students, 6 of them are $10 drop-ins at $60 per class, the others prepaid on the package plan.
- You are averaging $60 per class in drop-in clients, or $240 per month.

= $280 for the month.

Breakdown:

Average prepay 4 at $35 = $140

Drop-ins (6 at $10 x 4) = $240

Total Income = $380

Rent = $100

Balance $280. Owner's class pay and administrative fee. This is your pay, but don't forget you'll need to pay any expenses like music, sign-in sheets, taxes, etc. So you average $70 a class.

If you pay a sub one time at $25, your fee goes down to $255.

Space Rental Example #2

- You have 3 classes per week. Monday, Wednesday at 6 pm and Saturday at 10:00 am.
- You pay a flat fee of $250 to use the space three times a week per month.
- You offer a flat fee of $75 for unlimited classes which comes out to about approximately $6 per class.
- Drop in rate is $10 per class.
- Monthly calculations are represented by 4.3 weeks x 3 classes per week = 12.9 classes per month.
- Take $75 flat fee and divide by 12.9 average classes and you get $5.81 per class.
- Each month you have 4 people who pay $75 which = $350
- You have an average of 4 drop ins per class at $10 each (8 people usually come, average for a midsize town) =$40
- You have $40 drop ins for 12.9 classes a month =$516
- $350 for prepay

_____

= $868 per month.

You must pay rent of $250.

You net $618 per month, or about $47 a class (not bad). Now you will need to do subtract your advertising and other costs from this total.

Once you establish a clientele it will more likely work like this. The key is showing up and giving your best week in and week out. It takes time to build up a clientele. You must be patient and consistent.

Space Rental Example #3

Take the same numbers but use an average of 15 students. This would be an average for someone teaching a long time in a larger area, most likely. I've never seen class size stay consistent at 15 for very long in a medium to small town.

$75 per person for 7 people = $525
$10 per person at an average of 8 = $80
$80 drop-ins x 12.9 classes per month = $1,032
Total income for one month ($525 + $1032) = $1557
   - $250 rent

You net $1,307

Remember you will likely spend on advertising, props, copies, office supplie,s etc. Let's say that ends up costing you $157 a month. You still would clear $1,150 or $89.14 per class.

Private Lessons, Intensives (Events), Parties, and Corporate Yoga

In several of these instances, the teachers should have experience before embarking on taking private clients and teaching intensives. Only teach what you know and always remember that you'll never get ahead if your client suffers an injury.

Private Lessons

Prices for private lessons vary from $35 to $150, depending on the area. I am a yoga therapist and I live in a midsize rural area, so I only charge $50 to $75 per hour; however, if I lived in a metropolitan area I might charge double that. It is my mission to serve and to help people who need it, so I consider this when setting my fee. However, I also need to remember that if I set my fee too low, I may feel resentment.

The prices have gone down for private yoga sessions from what I can see since there is much more competition to drive down the price. So be mindful of what the going rate is in your area. New teachers will charge less and should be doing simple private classes like helping students understand the basics of yoga. More seasoned teachers can work with students who have special needs. Only teach what you know because you can do more harm than good if you take on a special needs client and you are not prepared for the task at hand.

Remember that studios and gyms will usually request 25% to 30% overhead to use their space for private lessons. On average, you can expect to make $25 to $100 for your time.

Intensives

I recommend that teachers who have not acquired E-RYT 200 status should not teach workshops. Workshops are generally taught for ongoing education, and teachers will show up expecting continuing education credit. If you want to share something you love, for instance a "Chakras and Yoga" class, then teach a 2-hour intensive. This is a great way to generate income doing something you are passionate about.

We used to offer intensives in my small-town yoga studio about every six weeks. The teacher made 70% and we would cross-market. I would put it on our Facebook page and website, and the teacher was encouraged to market his or her intensive on social media and otherwise as well. We would advertise the intensive, and I would help the teacher with the curriculum. Below is an example.

2-hour Intensive or Workshop Breakdown:
Timeline:
- First 30 minutes: Quick introductions and discussion on the topic. Quick bathroom break.

- Approximately 1 hour 15 minutes: Practice.
- Last 15 minutes: Q and A, any final thoughts, dismissal.

Charges:

- We might charge $20 per person, but you could easily charge upwards of $50 if you are in an upscale area. At $20, we might average 20 people, meaning the event brought in $400. The teacher made $280 and the studio made $120 for overhead, supplies, and administration. Again, charging depends on the area. In urban areas, you could easily double those figures.

Parties

Wedding showers and yoga parties are definitely in fashion. Generally, you are going to need a plan to market these. Here is how I did it.

For $30 per person, setting the minimum at 10 people, I provide space for 3 hours, a teacher, a Greek appetizer plate, cookies, hibiscus tea, and a hostess. I took care of set up and clean up.

- $300 for ten people paid up front.
- Teacher: $75
- Food and Paper Goods: $100
- Studio and Host (Owner): $125

Corporate Yoga

Today it is fairly common for sports teams, hospitals, colleges, and corporate offices to offer health and wellness programs to their employees. Corporate yoga can be great for the teacher because you are typically only responsible for showing up and teaching the class.

Here are some things to consider when going to interview with organizations:

- Be prepared to present on the benefits or yoga and sell yourself.
- Research the organization well and/or talk to any employees, if possible, to get a grasp on the organizational culture so that you can accurately describe how you can best serve them and demonstrate that you are conscientious and observant.
- Ask if the company or organization has a budget in mind before you quote them your prices. They may surprise you and offer more than you expected.
- Go in with your goal and your bottom line in mind. Again, the average that you can expect varies greatly, but what I am seeing in Arkansas is anywhere from $35 to $75 per class for the teacher. The average in my area is about $50 per class. If you over price it, they may decide to cut you out in a budget crunch. If you underprice it, you will feel resentment. Decide what your time is worth and work from there. If giving up your time for family or other activities for half a day or for two or three hours is worth $50, then you know your starting point.

Summing up Financials and Where to Teach

Most yoga teachers have a combination of things they do to make a living. Many people have full-time jobs and are very happy teaching one class per week at a studio and having access to taking yoga at the studio at no extra cost and/or getting discounts on retail at the studio. Some teachers want to teach full time and need to make a living. Many of these people will also have some other source of income. Keep in mind that it is challenging making a career out of yoga if you have no other source of income. The lifestyle is great; however, the tradeoff is you may have to live a simpler life if teaching yoga is your only income stream.

I often run into students who feel guilty about charging for yoga because they heard that yoga was free in India. In most cases that is not true. These rumors may stem from the fact that yoga students once worked for their practice, brought gifts of food like potatoes and onions, or worked in trade cleaning or doing chores. I myself barter as often as I can; however in modern life we need cash, pure and simple. The yoga teacher has bills to pay and the yoga student feels that they are getting their money's worth when they have a well-trained and capable teacher who is shaping them. Teaching yoga and taking yoga is an exchange of energy. There are real world expenses in doing just about every type of service.

Take a long look at yourself and your needs, and ask yourself questions before embarking on this journey. Teaching can be exhausting if you are only teaching and not caring for yourself in return. Look to Workbook questions for guidance on this subject.

Advertising and Marketing Ethically

I have seen many people open studios or start classes with the attitude that if you offer it they will come. This is not so. There is a huge market out there for yoga. There are classes at gyms, churches, studios, recreational centers, online, etc. How do you get people to come to your classes or business?

Establish the who, what, when, where, and cost:

The Who: It is imperative that you know who you are as a teacher and market yourself as such. You need to write down your credentials and experience and document any workshops and trainings you take. If you are an RYT 200 and you teach gentle classes, you will need to define that so people can know what to expect. Make sure to add contact information so students can get in touch with you for any questions and how to pay. Include your phone number, email, public Facebook page, and any other social media you utilize.

The What: Describe what you are teaching in about one to three sentences and make it very clear. "A hatha yoga class that is available to beginners. Focus is on the breath, gentle postures to relieve aches and pains, and mediation to calm the mind." If I as a consumer previously walked into a hot vinyasa class and did not like it, this tells me that you are offering something different that I could try. Be clear and specific.

What to Bring: Be clear about any details about what to wear (comfortable clothes you can move in), what to bring (a yoga mat), and anything else you need them to have or know before coming to class.

The When: Look to what is going on in your community. Most classes need to be offered between 5:30 a.m. and 7:30 a.m., then 8:15 a.m. to 11:00 a.m., and start back again between 4:15 p.m. and 8 p.m. In some cases, lunch classes go over, but often those are more difficult to fill. It really depends on your clientele and location. Avoid offering classes during times when people are traveling to work or school and home again. Think like a consumer. Put the time on your marketing materials and adhere to it closely, beginning and ending on time.

The Where: Describe your location with an address and possibly a picture of the entrance or the building and a map. It is also important that people know where to park.

The Cost: Include the cost of the class in simple terms, such as "4 weeks for $50, or $15 drop-in. Sessions start up every four weeks." Tell them what forms of payment you take such as cash, checks, or credit cards.

Marketing with a Host

If you are working in conjunction with a host, such as a church or dance studio, be clear up front about the expectations you each have in marketing the classes in exchange for fees. For instance, I rent space at a local art center. They have no obligation to market for me. I do all my own marketing through my Facebook, emails, and webpage. However, over the years we have started to cross-market in our advertising and it has been mutually beneficial for both of us.

In many cases if you are offering a class or intensive, both parties would add that information to their websites and social media, or distribute via email or fliers. Be clear up front to avoid problems. Ask, "*What are your expectations for marketing classes*?" This little piece of advice can save a lot of heartache.

When I owned my studio, I had a printed schedule, an online schedule, a website, a Facebook page, and we made announcements in class. I requested my teachers to make announcements, share the schedule, and market their classes on social media and in fliers if they chose to do so. We would also make a flier for special events that both the studio and the teacher shared.

Teachers who actively marketed their classes had a higher percentage of students more easily which led to higher pay and job satisfaction.

Fliers, Posters, Postcards, and Graphics

Fliers and postcards are a great asset in marketing. Those can be posted out in the world at community centers, in the studios or places you teach, health food stores, etc. They can also be posted on your social media and other online sources. Keep them simple, direct, and add some pretty graphics for an overall eye-catching poster. Make sure to include all the details of the who, what, where, when, and cost on the poster. Remember to add contact information. It is also a good idea to have a business card with your website, email, phone number, and credentials on it. You never know when you'll need to pull one out to share.

Marketing Budgets

No-Budget-too-Small

Most yoga teachers are not making a lot of money teaching yoga. Teaching yoga is much like being a musician: you get paid when you show up for work, not necessarily when you are honing your craft. It takes time to build a clientele, get experience, learn what you are good at, and learn what you don't like to teach.

So how do you get the word out? It isn't as hard as one might think. Making a flier is simple. It can be handmade and copied on a printer or made online with simple software like Microsoft Word. Using social media is probably the most productive and cheapest thing you can do to get people to your classes. I've had good success with targeted Facebook Ads for as little as $10. Post fliers in local businesses and nonprofits (get permission first), but especially leave a stack where you will be teaching. Post your fliers on Facebook and other forms of social media.

Some other free and simple ways of getting the word out are simply calling people you know and sending emails. Eblasts through MailChimp are free up to a certain number of recipients and are easy to format. Get on the phone and call everyone you know or send an email and invite them to your class. Good old word of mouth never hurts. You can offer incentives like two for the price of one for the first class to encourage people to come.

There are many free website services out there to use to build a simple website including all your information. I use Weebly.com and love it.

Medium Budgets

When you have a little more money, there are some other simple things you can add in to broaden your reach.

People still read the newspaper where I live. If I put an advertisement in my local paper every three months, I can get one "news brief" or "free announcement" as well during that ninety-day period. I will often run a $100 ad on a weekend when more people read the paper and then once every quarter to announce something big that we are doing or some sort of training one of our teachers has taken. Also, ask about bulk pricing as the cost goes down if you agree to advertise 6 times a year versus just calling when you need one ad. If you have never advertised then they will sometimes have a new customer package as well so be sure to ask what deals they offer. Being in the paper keeps you in the eye of the community, and builds recognition and goodwill for your brand.

The same concept goes for local magazines. You want to utilize magazines that are in the LOHAS market (Lifestyles of Health and Sustainability) when possible. For many years, I advertised with a magazine called *Natural Awakenings* once per month for about $150 and took out a quarterly news brief for free. If you do not have a magazine that is geared toward health, then look to "society" magazines. These are the magazines that feature local events and businesses. You will often see pictures of people in your local community in them. Everyone reads these as they are in every business waiting room in town. They are generally good investments if you are making enough to afford it. I would also suggest advertising during the months from January to March—generally the busy months for yoga. September to November can also be busy. Summers and holidays often slow down.

Social media advertising is another way to increase traffic. I had a bad experience with one major player in online advertising. However, I have had good experiences with "boosting" posts or targeted marketing with Facebook. You can choose your budget and target audience. You can spend as much or as little as you want to spend. I would recommend you talk to others before using this method and ask their experience. You don't want to give anyone permission to debit your credit card unless you are sure of the security safeguards, and beware of checking any auto-renewal boxes.

Larger Budgets

Radio and television advertising can be expensive, but can be a great way to get your name out. The cost for this type of marketing in my area averages somewhere around $300 per month or more, depending on the target area. It is important to know your market when advertising like this. If you are in a town of mostly young tech professionals, you will miss that market by booking a spot on the oldies but goodies radio station. On the other hand, if you are in a retirement community, you do want to be on that station if you are offering yoga for the senior population. If you have more money, you can take out bigger and more colorful print ads more often that will capture the eye of the consumer.

In summary, a good marketing plan will be varied and will cross-market in print, audio, and audio visual when available. You need to be keenly in touch with your brand and what you are offering before you begin marketing. Simple, clear, eye-catching marketing materials are very important. The estimated budget for marketing is usually somewhere between 5% and 10 % of the overall gross budget for a business. In saying that, I will tell you that I generally spend about 3% to 5% of my budget on marketing and use free marketing as much as possible.

Studio Location

Finding a good location can be tricky. I have seen many yoga studios in offbeat places do very well. There are many of ways to view this. If you are on a main street, you will deal with a lot of noise which can be distracting, but your visibility is high. If you are on a side street or off the beaten path you will want good directions and highly visible signage. A yoga studio is a destination business rather than a place where you get a lot of walk-in traffic. If someone gets frustrated trying to find you, they may not come for fear of being late for class.

If you can find a studio that has walkability, this is often a major plus. Two of my students have successful studios that are close to neighborhoods where people could easily walk from home to class.

In my situation, I had a brick and mortar building in a million-dollar location next to a popular big box store. Traffic also stopped in front of my studio at two stop lights. I invested a lot of money in signage facing both the store and the street. This was a wise use of my advertising budget. I was not in a walkable location, however.

In contrast, I live in a tourist town and I rent space in an art school and studio. I have purchased yard signs to put out when we are there. I'm also considering a bigger banner. There is another yoga studio a block away so I do not want people to get confused, but honestly that does happen a few times a month. In my advertising, I show a picture of the building I am in and tag it in my social media marketing. We are all very close and everyone is welcomed when they walk in the door. Since I have been teaching for sixteen years in the same community, we have a clientele that knows where to find us and through advertising in local media, social media, and website, we stay fairly full with eight to twenty plus students a week per class. Classes are full and we are content.

Business Ethics in the Yoga World

With the rise in the use of social media as a business platform, there seems to be a sea change in the world of people hiding behind a screen or rationalizing decisions since you can find someone to support nearly every decision, ethical or unethical, online these days.

A former employee said to me one day, "It is just business." My experiences have shaped me into the business woman I am today. There of course have been times when I made mistakes and learned from them and times when the things I choose to do turned out very well. Being in business is not always easy but it is easier when you know you are basing your actions on your values. Reviewing my own choices and witnessing the impact others' choices have had on them has had a great effect on the way I choose to conduct my business affairs. I strongly disagree with the statement "It's just business." These words are always a red flag to me, and a red flag also flies when others try to justify their actions with, "I have to make money, too." Separating oneself from ones business actions never seems to lead to good things.

We all know the golden rule: "Do unto others as you would have them do unto you." In yoga, we have the yamas and niyamas as guides for living ethical lives. These tenets can guide you dependably in life *and* in business. I recommend you read them often and become very self-aware. One of the most challenging things can be to trust that you can forgo temporary gain for doing the right thing and being able to face yourself in the mirror at the end of the day. Being ethical and making the right decisions even when it is difficult may in fact result in things like less income or notoriety. But leading with integrity and ethical practices will result in being able to sleep at night, will build your credibility, and will shape your brand. Ultimately, these could lead to more income and notoriety. Ultimately, you will profit from ethical behavior. You will also be a true "yogi" when you follow these time-tested philosophies.

Working for Others

As you start out, you will likely be working for a studio or health club. These are some things to carefully consider:

1. You are building a clientele, however that studio or gym is spending money on advertising to build their clientele as well. Their contact list is not your contact list. You should never contact students outside of the studio without the permission from the owner of the studio or gym. For example, it is not appropriate to send friend requests on Facebook to your students, but it is okay for them to send you a friend request to you and you accept it. You should not solicit students. Never take a contact list with you or copy it without permission when you leave a job or employer. You can be sued for doing so.

2. If you build or design fliers, websites, etc., for a studio owner or employer, and are paid to do so, your work product is the legal property of the employer who has hired you to do the work. If you copy sign-in sheets, waivers, fliers, etc., you could be sued for stealing trade secrets or intellectual property. It is helpful to develop relationships with a community of seasoned yoga teachers who will gladly share forms and other useful information with you in an ethical way.

3. So what do you do if you want to leave an employer and venture out on your own? First, quit your job before you start the new one or start building the new job officially. You should do your own advertising and let the clients find you. NEVER discuss your leaving

with the students in the location of your present job without the consent of your supervisor. When I left a large nonprofit, I had many students and many had followed me there. I did not speak of leaving. I gave my two-week notice and told my boss at the time that I did not think it was a good idea for me to continue to teach because it would put pressure on me in the classroom to discuss where I was going. I asked to be taken off the floor and to continue only my administrative duties. I officially left my job at the nonprofit before I announced publicly through my website, Facebook, and on social media that I was opening a studio. I did not contact any students in any form to let them know where I was going even though some of them had followed me for years. If you stay in the same community, then the ones that want to will find you. Many came to me for classes but many did not because the nonprofit offered classes at a much-reduced price. Be aware that having many students at one location doesn't mean they will follow you to a new location. There are many decisions that clients make when choosing yoga, and price and location can be huge factors.

4. When posting your classes on social media here are some of the courtesy dos and don'ts: it is fine to say "Come see me at 9:00 a.m. at XYZ yoga studio for a gentle yoga class." It is okay to post on XYZ yoga studio page as well about your class. It is not ethical or appropriate to post, "Come see me at 9:00 am XYZ yoga studio, and at Ginny's gym at 11:30 for restorative yoga." Why might this be a problem? Because those places are paying you to work for them and you are cross-marketing yourself in a post with both of their names in it. That studio or gym has invested more than just paying you. They have invested in pulling students into your classes in their business through expensive marketing. Also, they may not want to be associated with one another for reasons unbeknownst to you and it is not appropriate for you to decide to pair them together. It is best and most considerate to do separate post.

5. When working for more than one business, marketing yourself can be tricky. When you are in the location where you are teaching your classes and someone asks you where else you teach, I advise trying to avoid that conversation unless you teach in places that are noncompetitive. When I was in this position, **I generally tried not to work for two competing businesses.** I worked for a local community college and a local health club which were not in competition with one another. As a studio owner, dealing with this was a huge source of frustration. When I worked in administration for a large nonprofit it was very clear to me that I was not to hire people who worked for the competition unless we were desperate for teachers. This is not discussed much in the world of yoga. Studios generally do not want to hire teachers who work regularly for other studios that are in the same vicinity and market to the same population. It is not the same with a sub, as this is not a permanent position, though studios often use their own people to sub before they will reach out to other contractors. I am not saying this never happens, what I am saying is from my experience studio owners and school owners will discuss this between themselves but not with teachers. They may hire teachers who work for competitors however it is not usually something they generally like to do.

6. Market who and what you are. It is important to know what the competition is doing. In yoga, many people don't like the word competition. It is often treated like a dirty word as if something is wrong with us for even discussing that it exists. But it does exist and there are a lot of people sticking their heads in the sand to avoid talking about it. Many people are trying to say it is collaboration, not competition. I'm here to tell you that is not the case most of the time. *So what is the difference between competition and collaboration?* Collaboration looks like this. On May 1st every year all the yoga studios in town give away 20% of their profits to the Humane Society and they have a big marketing campaign. The Humane Society has a website that lists all studios participating. Collaboration is offering a community event where the studios come together to teach an event like "Yoga Day" at a park. On the other hand, competition is when two or more places are competing for the same population to come to their studio for classes, events, workshops, etc. *How do we ethically compete?* First, do not degrade your competition or talk negatively about them. Focus on what you do and what your specialties are, rather than trying to degrade their offerings. I have been around the yoga community a long time and I see it all the time. I or one of my sister studios (or teachers) will offer something unique that came from their own experience and within two months, the competition is offering the same thing. That is the nature of capitalism. However, there is a better way. **Be who you are.** Do what is natural and authentic for you and capitalize on it. That is the only way you will be able to sustain it. I teach a regular beginner-friendly class that is therapeutic in nature. I promote on my experience, credentials, and the nature of what I do as well as the fact that we are community-oriented and welcoming. I do not even know the schedule of the studio down the street from me. I do keep up with what others are charging and so forth, but I focus on what I am doing and what I do well. And more importantly, I look at what the community needs and is asking for and match my gifts with that. When you serve, and are in service to others in an authentic way, people will come.

Section 8: The Yoga Lifestyle

What does it mean to live a yoga lifestyle? It is not about the clothes you wear, the music you listen to, or the amount of asana you practice. So then, what is it? The answer to that question is not so easy. As I write this book I have had a consciously active life as a yogi for over two thirds of my life. Here is what I have gathered from all those years of study and practice.

Yoga is, essentially, in the eye of the practitioner. Many may think that to be a yogi you must be vegan, wear only certain styles of clothing, ride a bike, practice pranayama, asana, and meditation every day, and live a very austere life. Yoga is just not that simple, nor does it easily fit in a box. In my world view, a person who lives a yoga lifestyle follows the eight limbs of yoga, especially following the yamas and the niyamas. However, each person will differ on how they interpret these based on their views and experiences. Yoga is a mind-body practice that teaches us to find balance, so for me, any practice that brings the mind and body together in an effort to achieve balance in a healthy way is yoga. In the Western world, the state of balance in the body is known as homeostasis. For some, the practice of karma yoga or selfless service may be their yoga. For others, walking and worshiping may be their yoga. Every day that you practice being mindful you are practicing yoga. Every time you get knocked off center and you go to your mat you are practicing yoga. Every time you get emotionally pulled out of balance and you sit and examine your thoughts and feelings and objectively look at your actions, you practice yoga. When you read spiritual texts, donate your time, help another, live by faith, consciously purchase, consciously consider your actions, you are practicing yoga. Life itself is like a pendulum; it swings to the left and the right and it finds balance in the center. What we do to find that balance is yoga. When we are swinging wildly about, we need yoga. If you are living a life of excess, or are in pain, the practice of yoga can help.

Yoga itself is ever-evolving, forming, and reforming, especially the asana practice. What doesn't change are the basics—the eight limbs and the tenets of yoga. Within the vastness of yoga, should we choose to practice it, we all have to find our own way. Fortunately, though, there are teachers and guides to help us, even as we ourselves become teachers and guides.

Let me give an example from my experience as a Yoga Therapist. For many years, I taught classes and private yoga along with workshops and teacher trainings. Over and over I saw people come to the mat for physical reasons only to have emotional reactions to the practice. In my private practice and with the school I would often have students come to me on the verge of breakdown because they were unsure of how and why yoga was changing them. They experienced feelings, flashbacks, or even movement in their lives they were not prepared for. I would help the best I could by offering from my own experience of how yoga helped me. The problem was I carried all the weight of those people's problems home with me at night. Over time, I decided I would find a coaching program to help me with some communication tools to empower these people who were approaching me, and to absorb some of that weight and transfer the energy into something meaningful. I went through a coaching course and it transformed the way I teach.

I share this with you only as a guide. These methods should only be used by experienced teachers, social workers, and trained yoga therapists. However, you are welcome to incorporate some of these methods in your teaching. That being said, I implore you to not teach yoga therapy without serious experience in your field. I am sharing this information as a Certified Yoga Therapist and Stress Management Specialist.

Teaching Tips:
First, I ask a series of questions to lead the person on a quest of self-discovery. *What hurts? Has your doctor told you not to do any type of movement or exercise? Have you been released to practice yoga? Do you have a diagnosis? What are your obstacles, strengths, and weaknesses? What's working and what's not working?* Through coaching methods, I find out what's going on. I am not giving advice here, simply asking questions to help me plan a private session for the client.

I explain some principles of yoga to the student and how the practice will help them student through pranayama, asana, positive thinking, affirmations, and meditation. Then I design and lead them through these steps which I organize around what they have told me. We set up attainable goals and meet several times with a deadline.

I developed this type of yoga therapy based on a combination of personal experiences. Generally, in the field of private yoga or yoga therapy, it may look like this. Client A comes to you with a bulging disc. You design an asana practice for bulging disc with some breath work and meditation to help with relaxation. Then, you teach it to the client, and send them home with the practice. They come every week for six weeks and you monitor the progress and make needed changes. If that is all the client desires, that is perfectly fine.

Living a Happy Life with Yoga

I used to believe that contentment was the best we could hope for. There would be moments of happiness along the way but each day would likely be good if we were just content. Since 2011, I have been adhering to some strict guidelines for self-care. This approach has made all the difference for me in understanding that we can have happiness over contentment more often when we self-care. *You know what?* I am happy. I am happy every day, not all day long, but each day I find moments of happiness. Sure, I get upset, angry, and have bad days, but even so, every day I find something to be happy about. I can advise you whole-heartedly to not settle for contentment when you can have happiness. It is within reach; it is inside you right now. It takes work, but the good news is the work is wonderful and fun! Reach inside.

Personal Story:
My Yoga Lifestyle

Each week I walk, do a little strength training, and practice yoga. I try to avoid negative media and to limit time spent on social media and anything with electronic screens—phones, televisions, computers, etc. I make a point to get out in nature daily or at least weekly, having learned there is no better way to balance myself than to be by water and greenery. Each day when a negative thought comes up, I try to turn it into something positive. For instance, when my kid leaves the light on for the billionth time, I do say something to them, but instead of only focusing on the high electricity bill, I try to give thanks that I have that problem when so many people live without their basic needs being met. I live in the real world of challenges and times of suffering, but I don't let my mind give too much energy to negative thinking. When challenges come along I think through them carefully, come up with a plan to deal with them, and trust myself to know what is best. And when life throws me a terribly painful situation, I go to yoga classes or practice at home, meditate, talk to people I love, and take extra good care of myself. I try to extend myself deep wells of self-compassion because regardless of what I know or my training, I am still an imperfect human being who makes mistakes. I may ask for advice, but ultimately I gauge my own feelings first and must trust myself to know what is best for me. This is key. You must trust yourself. Others may give good advice and you should listen, but at the end of the day you need to know if that advice fits you or not. Take your time and it will come.

Advice from My Decades as a Yogini

Focus on your strengths. Know what you are good at. Notice what you do not enjoy or feel confident in and find a solution to handle it. I am not good with tools, so I ask my fiancé to do that kind of work for me or I hire someone. Recently I needed some help marketing, so I hired someone to help me rewrite a resume and guide me on print marketing. I saved more than I spent by recognizing that I couldn't do it all. Each day, do healthy things like walking and sitting on your porch swing. Schedule three important tasks each day and do them, but also take a day or two off each week. When you need to stop and rest, do so. If you feel sick, your best will be different from a day when you have a lot of energy. Give yourself a break. Listen to your body. Drink lots of water. Eat healthy meals. Exercise. Schedule your time wisely. Be with positive people. Smile. Be kind. Be of service. Be empathetic. Be compassionate. Compliment yourself, your family, and others. Say "no" when you need to. Say "yes" when you want to. Sometimes you must compromise; however, do not make a habit or doing things out of guilt and learn to recognize codependent behavior. It is one thing to be kind, but be careful of enabling others to rely on you to meet their needs. If someone can do something for themselves, do not do it for them unless they need it or you simply want to do something loving for someone. Recognize the difference. I learned this from raising four kids, including two with special needs. On the other hand, don't be self-involved. When you do something think about the other person and ask why you are doing what you are doing. Be genuine and authentic in your giving and receiving in life.

Do well, make good choices, and be kind to yourself and others. Take care of yourself now rather than waiting until you are older. The time is now to figure out what self-care means. Balance this with service to others. Recognize that for every action there is a reaction. Energy out equals what you will get in return. If you put healthy and balanced love into a relationship, you will likely get love in return. If you don't, prepare yourself and move on without fear. Work hard and you will be paid well. Be a good friend and you will have good friends. Listen to your instincts. Trust your intuition. When things are not working, let go. Learn to know, learn to hear, learn to just be in your blissful, natural state of peace. Remember, you are the lotus.

Section 9: Sample Classes and Guidelines

Sample Class

Opening meditation or intention: Look to your mediation books or study guided imagery. Set the intention with a reading or a suggestion like, *"Now you are here on your mat. Let the outside world go, and set an intention to bring your focus back to what is happening on your mat today."*

Class Beginning

- **Pranayama**. Three-part breathing, focused breathing, alternate nostril breathing, or ujjayi for three to five breaths.

- **Warming Up the Body**. Opening postures and joint loosening.

- **Half Sun Salute**. See page 58.

Class Middle

- **Full Sun Salute**. See page 58. I generally put backbends here if you are building them into a class, at the point where you would do cobra. This is a good place as it flows more naturally, or you can put them right after the warm up and then go to child's pose, up to down dog, and up to your standing poses.

- **Choose Postures and Sequence**. Standing postures, balancing postures, seated postures, seated twists, reclined postures, and inversions. Always counter the spine with a bridge, reclined spinal twist, and knees to chest.

Class End

- **Shavasana**.

- **Namaste**. *"The light (divine) in me recognizes the light in you."* Often you will hear only "Namaste," at the end of class. In other traditions, you may hear "Om, Shanti, Shanti, Shanti, Om," then "Namaste." Choose what you are comfortable with.

Sample Class — *Illustrated Example*

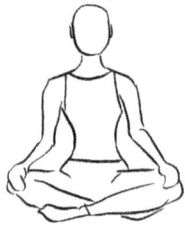 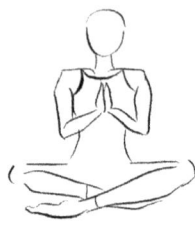 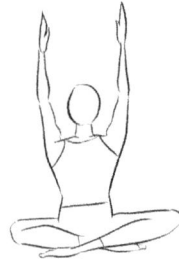 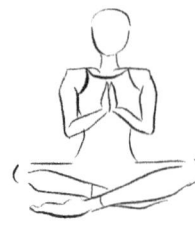 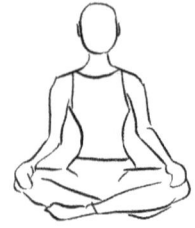

(Inhale)   (Exhale)

Easy Pose with arm movements and breath, repeat x3

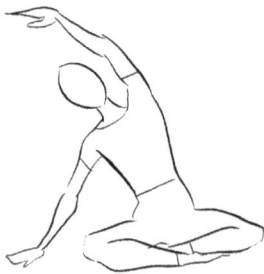 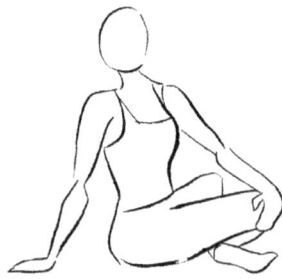 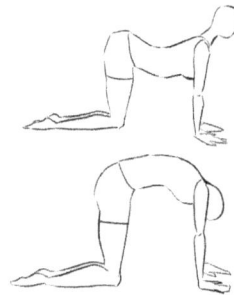 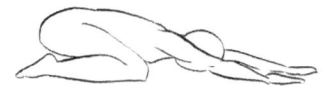

Side Lean
L/R

Seated Twist
L/R

Cow Cat

Child's Pose

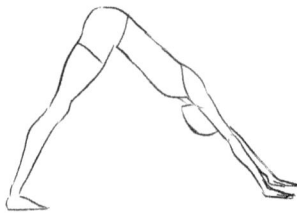 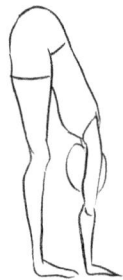 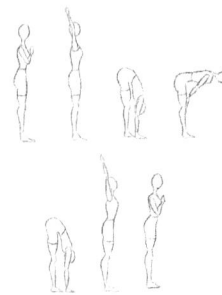 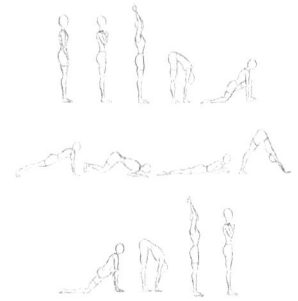

Downward
Facing Dog

Standing
Forward Fold

1/2 Sun Salute

Full Sun Salute

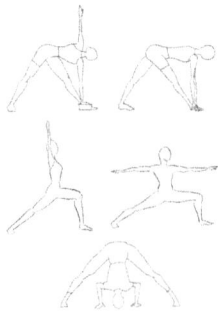 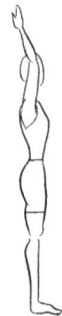 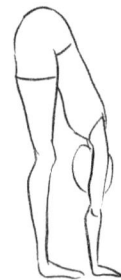 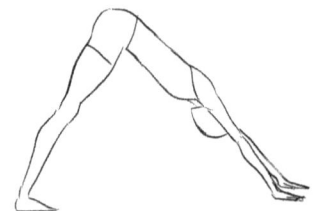

Triangle, Pyramid,
Warrior 1, Warrior 2,
Wide-Legged Forward Fold
*Repeat on both sides

Extended
Mountain

Standing
Forward Fold

Down Dog

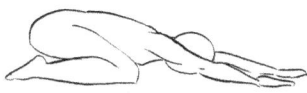

Child's Pose

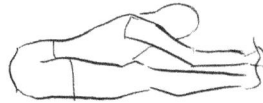

Seated
Forward Fold

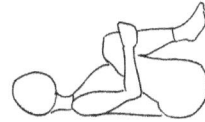

Knees to Chest

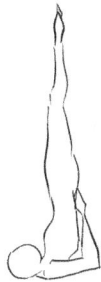

Shoulder Stand

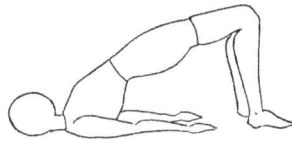

Bridge

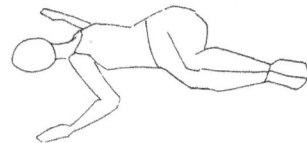

Reclined Twist
L/R

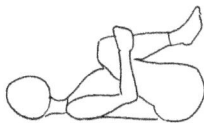

Knees to Chest

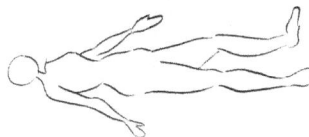

Corpse
(Shavasana)

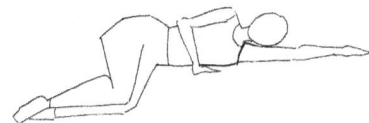

Seed / Rescue

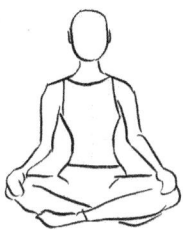 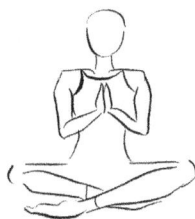 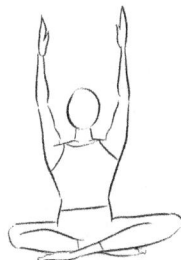 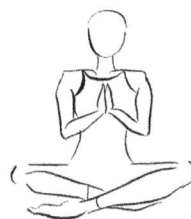 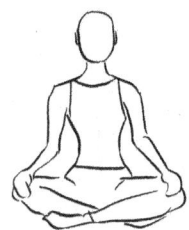

(Inhale)   (Exhale)

Back to Easy Pose with arm movements and breath, repeat x3

Sample Class 2 - *Photo Example*

Gentle Balanced Practice

This practice is great for back pain and stress relief. You will need a chair, pillow, and yoga mat. Expect the practice to last approximately 45 minutes to an hour when each pose is held for three to five breaths, including a ten minute Shavasana.

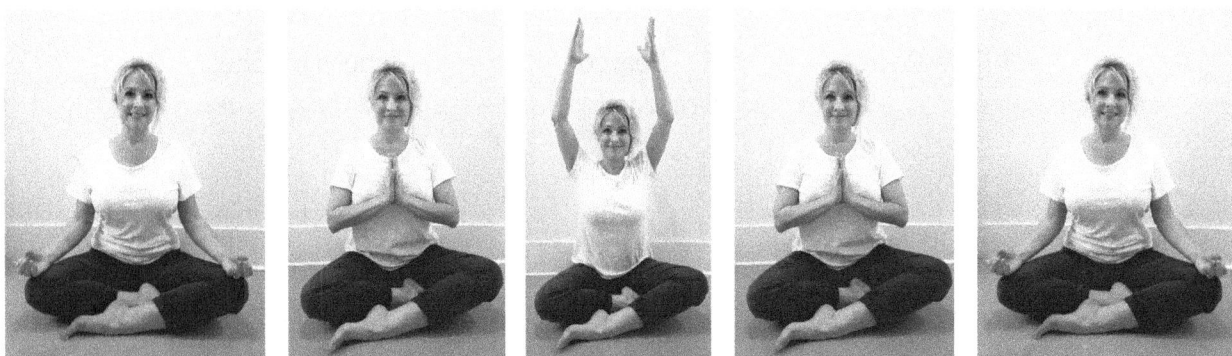

Easy Pose with arm movements and breath, repeat x3

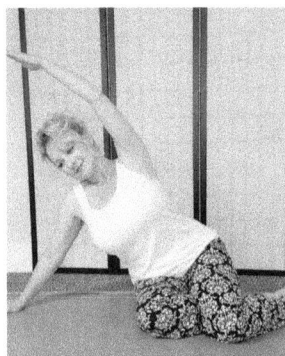

Seated Side Lean
L/R

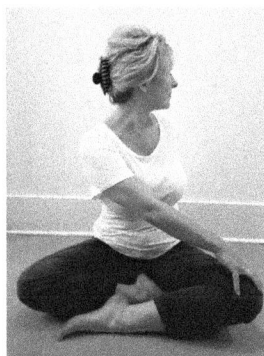

Seated Twist
L / R

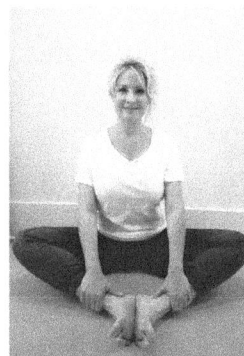

Cobbler

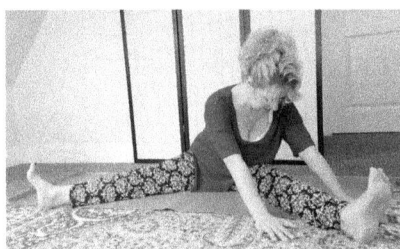

Seated Wide Leg
Forward Fold L/R

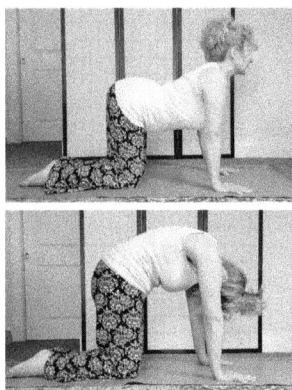

Cow/ Cat

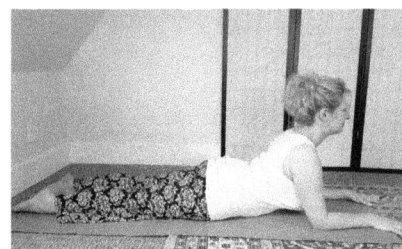

Sphinx

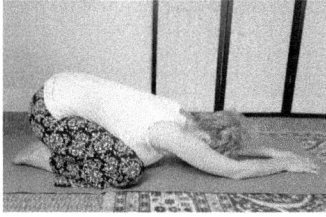

Child's Pose

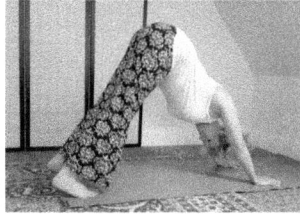

Downward
Facing Dog

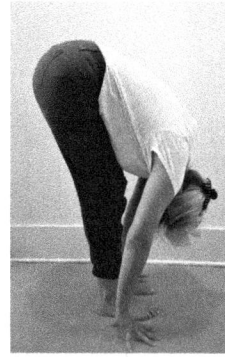

Standing
Forward Fold

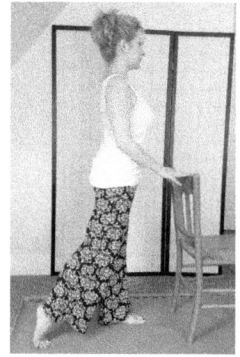

Standing Locust
L/R

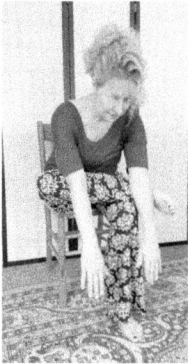

Seated Hip Fold* -
Figure 4, thread the
needle L/R

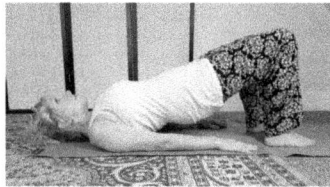

Bridge

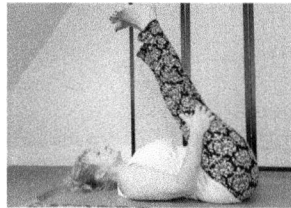

Reclined
Leg Stretch

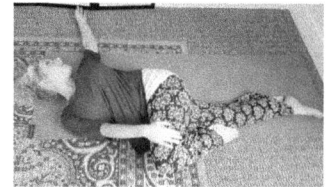

Reclined Twist
L/R

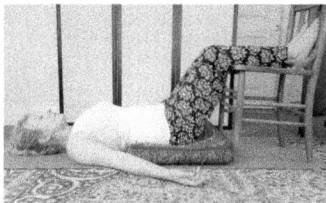

Modified Shoulder
Stand

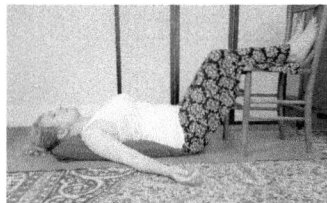

Fish

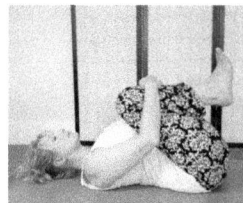

Knees to Chest

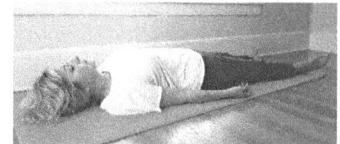

Shavasana

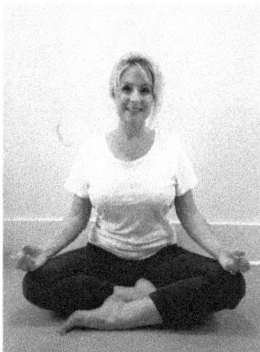

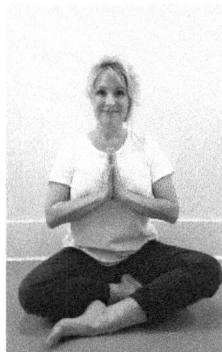

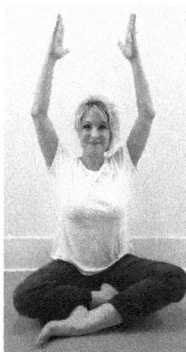

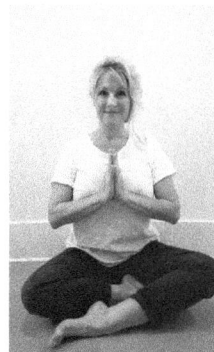

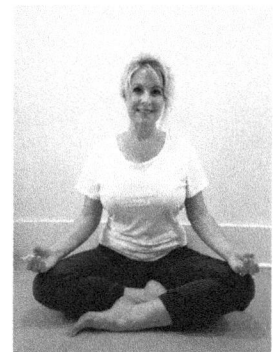

Easy Pose with arm movements and breath, repeat x3

Bibliography

Books

Beattie, Melody. *Journey to the Heart: Daily Meditations on the Path to Freeing Your Soul.* San Francisco, CA: HarperSanFrancisco, 1996. Print.

Beattie, Melody. *The Language of Letting Go.* Center City, MN: Hazelden, 1990. Print.

Bell, Baxter, and Nina Zolotow. *Yoga for Healthy Aging: A Guide to Lifelong Well-Being.* Boulder: Shambhala, 2017. Print.

Birch, Beryl Bender, and Nicholas DeSciose. *Power Yoga: The Total Strength and Flexibility Workout.* New York: Simon & Schuster, 1995. Print.

Fabian, Karen. *Stretched: Build Your Yoga Business, Grow Your Teaching Techniques.* Createspace Independent Platform, 2014. Print.

Gates, Rolf, and Katrina Kenison. *Meditations from the Mat: Daily Reflections on the Path of Yoga.* New York: Anchor, 2002. Print.

Herrington, Sarah. *Yoga (Idiot's Guides).* 1st ed. INpolis, IN: Alpha, A Member of Penguin Group (USA), 2013. Print.

Iyengar, B. K. S. *Light on Yoga: Yoga Dipika.* New York: Random House, 1994. Print.

Kappmeier, Kathy Lee, and Diane M. Ambrosini. *Instructing Hatha Yoga.* Champaign, IL: Human Kinetics, 2006. Print.

Mitchell, Stephen. *Bhagavad Gita: A New Translation.* New York: Three Rivers, 2006. Print.

Page, Joseph Le, and Lilian Le Page. *Yoga Teacher's Toolbox.* Shelby, NC: Integrative Yoga Therapy, 2005. Print.

Patañjali, and Alistair Shearer. *The Yoga Sūtras of Patañjali.* New York: Bell Tower, 2002. Print.

Payne, Larry, Terra Gold, and Eden Goldman. *Yoga Therapy & Integrative Medicine: Where Ancient Science Meets Modern Medicine.* Laguna Beach: Basic Health Publications, 2015. Print.

Payne, Larry. *Yoga For Dummies, 3rd Edition.* N.p.: John Wiley & Sons, 2014. Print.

Schiffmann, Erich. *Yoga: The Spirit and Practice of Moving into Stillness.* New York: Pocket, 1996. Print.

Stryker, Rod. *The Four Desires: Creating a Life of Purpose, Happiness, Prosperity, and Freedom.* New York: Delacorte, 2011. Print.

Ancient Texts

Hatha Yoiga Pradipka, Svāmi Svātmārāma.

Yoga Korunta, Vama Rishi.

The Upishands.

The Vedas.

Films

Ashtanga, NY - A Yoga Documentary. Dir. Caroline Laskow and Mary Wigmore. Perf. Willem Defoe and Regina French. First Run Features, 2014.

AWAKE: The Life of Yoganda. Dir. Paola Di Florio and Lisa Leeman. Perf. George Harrison and Anupam Kher. Alive Mind, 2014.

Breath of the Gods. Dir. Jan Schmidt-Garre. Perf. B.K.S. Iyengar, Patabhi Jois, and T. Krishnamacharya. PARS Media, 2012.

Enlighten Up! Dir. Kate Churchill. Perf. B.K.S. Iyengar and Pattabhi Jois. Docurama, 2009.

Websites

Ananda: Meditation, Yoga, Community, Teachings of Paramhansa Yoganda. Ananda Sangha Worldwide, Web. <www.ananda.org>.

Centre for Yoga Studies | The Art of Personal Sadhana. Paul Harvey, Web. <www.yogastudies.org>.

City-Data.com. Advameg, Inc., Web. <www.city-data.com/>.

Diffen - Compare Anything. Diffen. Discern. Decide. Diffen LLC, Web. <www.diffen.com>.

Dr. Melissa West. Melissa West, Web. <www.melissawest.com>.

Held, Lisa Elaine. "The Journey of Alan Finger, A Yoga Master's Master." *Wellandgood.com*. Well+Good LLC, 15 May 2013. Web. <www.wellandgood.com/good-sweat/alan-finger-yoga-master/>.

Lilias Yoga. Lilias M. Folan, Web. <http://www.liliasyoga.com/>.

Many Paths, One Yoga Alliance. Yoga Alliance, Web. <www.yogaalliance.org>.

Sivananda.org. The International Sivananda Yoga Vedanta Centres, Web. <www.sivananda.org/>.

Swami Satchidananda, Founder of Integral Yoga. Satchidananda Ashram - Yogaville, Web. <swamisatchidananda.org/>.

The International Association of Yoga Therapists: Bridging Yoga and Healthcare. The International Association of Yoga Therapists, Web. <www.iayt.org>.

Traditional Yoga and Meditation of the Himalayan Masters. Swami Jnaneshvara Bharati, Web. <www.swamij.com>.

Trieger, Rita. "Interview with John Kepner." *LA Yoga Magazine*. Bliss Network, LLC, 13 June 2013. Web. < www.layoga.com/practice/yoga-therapy/interview-with-john-kepner/>

Trulia: Real Estate Listings, Homes For Sale, Housing Data. Zillow Group, Web. <www.trulia.com/>.

Walden (Author), Patricia. "Yoga for Beginners: With Patricia Walden." *Yoga Journal*. Cruz Bay Publishing, Inc. Web.

Yoga Journal. Cruz Bay Publishing, Inc., Web. <www.yogajournal.com>.

Television

Folan, Lilias M. *Lilias, Yoga and You*. PBS. Cincinnati, Ohio. Television.

The Mud & The Lotus

A Workbook for Students of Yoga

Workbook Key appears on page 197.

How to use *The Mud & The Lotus: A Workbook for Students of Yoga*
As you read or after you complete your reading of *The Mud & The Lotus: A Guide for Students of Yoga*, you may reinforce its concepts through use of this workbook. It will be useful for teacher training, book-club-type study, or simply to holistically broaden one's knowledge of yoga. Its sections and contents correspond with the sections and contents of the Guide. If you run out of space as you answer questions, there are blank pages at the end of the workbook that you may use or feel free to extend your writings to your own notebooks or journals.

Section 1: Overview

What is Yoga?

Directions: Use the words below to fill in the blanks.

- bind
- unite
- yoke
- yogi

- yogis
- yogini
- yuj

1. The word yoga means to _____ or _____ together.

2. The root word of yoga is _____, which means to _____ together.

3. Those who practice yoga are called _____. A female who does yoga is called a _____ and a male who does yoga is called a _____.

4. Why might people be drawn to start a yoga practice?

The Eight Limbs of Yoga

Directions: Define each limb and/or its subcategory.

1. **Yamas** —

   Ahimsa —

   Satya —

   Asteya —

   Brahmacharaya —

   Aparigraha —

2. **Niyamas** —

   Saucha —

   Santosha —

Tapas —

Svadhyaya —

Ishvara Pranidhana —

3. **Asana** —

4. **Pranayama** —

5. **Pratyahara** —

6. **Dharana** —

7. **Dhyana** —

8. **Samadhi** —

Types of Yoga

Directions: Define the types of yoga listed below.

Karma —

Bhakti —

Jnana —

Tantra —

Mantra —

Raja —

Hatha —

The Five Points of Yoga

Swami Vishnudevananda condensed the essence of the yoga teachings into five principles for physical and mental health as well as spiritual growth. This is often helpful to new students to introduce them into a basic understanding of a yoga lifestyle.

Below list the five principals and define them:

1.

2.

3.

4.

5.

A Brief and Basic History of Yoga

Directions: Use the words below to fill in the blanks.

- Classical Period
- Debate
- Lifestyle
- Modern Period
- Post-Classical Period

- Pre-Classical Yoga
- Truths
- Veda
- Vedas
- Vedic Yoga Period

1. Yoga is a _____, not a religion.

2. There is much _____on how old yoga is.

3. The _____was from roughly 2000 to 1000 BCE. The _____are among the world's oldest sacred texts, and the oldest scriptures of Hinduism, written in Sanskrit. They are said to have been created by sages following long periods of meditation. _____means "knowledge" in Sanskrit.

4. The _____ Period is marked by the Upishads and the Bhagavad Gita.

5. During the _____ of Yoga, Pantajali wrote the Yoga Sutras, which described the 8 limbs of yoga. It includes 195 aphorisms, or _____, offering guidelines for a meaningful and purposeful life.

6. During the _____, emphasis shifted to living in the present and Swami Swatmarama composed the Hatha Yoga Pradipika, integrating the physical disciplines of hatha yoga with the spiritual goals of meditation.

7. During the _____, beginning in the late 19th and early 20th centuries, hatha yoga rises in popularity and there is an even greater focus on the physical body, and the connection of prana and the mind.

Directions: Match the words below with their appropriate definition.

- Bhagavad Gita
- Hatha Yoga Pradipika
- Upanishads
- Sutras

_____ Written between 800 and 500 BCE during the Pre-Classical Period, a collection of more than 200 sacred Sanskrit writings containing some of the central philosophical concepts of Hinduism. (Some of these concepts are shared with Buddhism, Jainism, and other religions.) They emphasized sacrifice of the ego through self-knowledge, action (karma yoga), and wisdom (jnana yoga).

_____ Translated "Lord's Song," tells the story of a warrior prince named Arjuna who confronts a moral dilemma and is led to a better understanding through the intercession of the god Krishna. It addresses the principles of karma (generous actions), bhakti (caring dedication), and jnana (knowledge), corresponding to the branches of yoga.

_____ Written during the Classical Period of yoga, this was the first systematic presentation of yoga. It described the eight-fold path or eight limbs of yoga, which were intended to be memorized. It describes the thread of the "lower self" joining together with the universal "higher self." Its aphorisms, or truths, are divided into four areas: concentration, practice, progressing, and liberation.

_____ Composed during the 15th Century by Swami Swatmarama, this text remains one of the most outstanding authorities on hatha yoga. Some of the original yoga postures are first laid out in this text, and its primary goal was illuminating the physical disciplines and practices of hatha yoga as integrated with higher spiritual goals of meditation.

Yoga Masters of India

Directions: Define these terms as you understand them and share when they may be used.

Guru:

Ji:

Swami:

Directions: Share some important facts about each teacher.

Sri T. Krishnamacharya —

K. Pattabhi Jois —

B.K.S. Iyengar —

Desikachar —

A.G. Mohan —

Swami Satchidananda —

Paramahansa Yogananda —

Modern Day Yoga Teachers

Directions: Share some important facts about each teacher, noting the style of yoga with which they are associated.

Erich Shiffman —

Lillias Folan —

Judith Hanson Lasiter —

Bikram Choudhury —

John Friend —

Larry Payne —

David Life and Sharon Gannon —

Baron Baptiste —

Bereyl Bender Birch —

Bernie Clark —

Anna Forest —

Rodney Yee —

Rolf Gates —

Seane Corn —

Shiva Rea —

Patricia Walden —

Gary Kraftsow —

John Kepner —

Rod Stryker —

Nikki Myers —

Dr. Baxter Bell —

Section 2: The Practice of Teaching

Credentialing

State Licenses

Directions: Use the words below to fill in the blanks.

- licensed
- not
- require

1. There are several states which _____ yoga schools to be licensed.

2. Arkansas does _____ license yoga schools.*

3. Yoga teachers are not _____ by the state in Arkansas.*

4. *(If not in Arkansas, look online to determine and circle.) The state in which I live or will teach does/does not license yoga schools and does/does not require that teachers be licensed.

Yoga Alliance

Directions: Use the words below to fill in the blanks.

- certificate
- credentialing
- nonprofit

1. Yoga Alliance is the largest _____ agency of yoga teachers.

2. Yoga Alliance is a _____ that sets standards for yoga schools and yoga teachers.

3. All accredited schools issue a _____ of completion and then the student may register with Yoga Alliance should they choose to do so.

Yoga Alliance School Designations

Directions: Match the program to its defining characteristics.

- 200 R.Y.S.
- 300 R.Y.S.
- 500 R.Y.S.
- R.C.Y.S.
- R.P.Y.S.
- Y.A.C.E.P.

_____ (Registered Yoga School at the 200 hour level). The program has an accumulation of 200 hours to graduate.

_____ (Registered Yoga School at the 300 hour level) 300 hour programs are set for students who have already attended a 200 hour program.

_____ (Registered Yoga School at the 500 hour level). This program is a full 500 hour program and students will qualify for a 500 R.Y.T. upon graduation.

_____ (Registered Children's Yoga School). A 95 hour curriculum that is geared towards teaching children. To register with Yoga Alliance one must first complete a 200 hour R.Y.S. to be able to obtain a registration for RCYT.

_____ (Registered Prenatal Yoga School) A 95 hour curriculum that is geared towards teacher pregnant and postnatal women. To register with Yoga Alliance one must first complete a 200 hour R.Y.S. to be able to obtain a registration as RPYT.

_____ (Yoga Alliance Continuing Education Provider) A new credential available to educators who are approved to provide continuing education to yoga teachers who are Registered with Yoga Alliance.

Yoga Alliance Teacher Designations

Directions: Match the program to its defining characteristics.

- E.R.Y.T. 200
- R.Y.T. 200
- R.C.Y.T.
- R.P.Y.T.
- R.Y.T.500
- E.R.Y.T. 500

_____ Must complete an accredited 200 R.Y.S. program. Must maintain continuing education every three years to keep registration current.

_____ An R.Y.T. 200 who has a minimum of 2 years teaching experience as well as 1,000 hours teaching in the classroom.

_____ Must complete a 200 and a 300 or a 500 hour accredited program. Must teach 100 hours since completing the program to apply for a 500 R.Y.T.

_____ Must have taught for a minimum of 4 years and have a minimum of 2000 hours teaching since receiving a 200 or 500 hour designation. 500 of those hours must be after receiving a 500 hour designation.

_____ Must be an R.Y.T. 200 in addition to completing an accredited R.Y.C.S. program.

_____ Must complete an R.Y.T. 200 program in addition to completing an accredited R.P.Y.T. program.

International Association of Yoga Therapists (I.A.Y.T.)

What does I.A.Y.T. do?

What is the credential given to yoga therapist?

What are the requirements to register as a yoga therapist with IAYT? *You may look on IAYT.org for more info.

Structuring a Class: The Bell Curve Method

Directions: Use the words below to fill in the blanks.

- backward bending
- beginning
- Bell Curve
- middle
- end
- forward bending
- lateral left/right
- twisting left/right
- forward bends and twists
- back bends and twists
- body
- mind

1. All styles of yoga vary somewhat in class structure. The best method we have found is the _____method. It has a _____, _____, and an _____.

2. The six directions of the spine are:

   1.

   2.

   3/4.

   5/6.

3. Back bends are balanced by _____.

4. Forward bends are balanced by _____.

5. Always balance every pose for physical and energetic reasons to keep the _____ and _____ balanced.

Directions: Use the words below to fill in the blanks.

- heart
- twist
- inversions
- props

- medical conditions
- introduce
- at home

1. Always _____ yourself to the students.

2. Tell them what _____ they will need.

3. Ask about any _____ prior to class and always have them sign a waiver before class starts.

4. Make them feel _____.

5. Students who have medical conditions such as glaucoma, high blood pressure, retinopathy, dizziness, or if they are pregnant should not be put in poses where the head is below the _____ (inversions). Pregnant students need to avoid deep _____ and should never be allowed to do extreme _____ like headstand or shoulder stand.

What does Namaste mean?

What does Shanti mean?

What's the significance of Om?

Permission Language

What is Permission Language?

Give some examples of Permission language as related to asana. For example, what alternative might you offer in forward fold for those who are curvy?

You're teaching alternate nostril breathing. You have a student with asthma who is not comfortable with this type of breathing. What permission language could you offer?

Music

Discuss this benefits and drawbacks of using music. What are some considerations before using music in yoga class?

How might music be utilized appropriately in a yoga class?

Styles of Yoga

Directions: Use the words below to fill in the blanks.
- stealing
- Hatha Yoga
- trademarked
- certified
- inspired by

1. There is a difference between styles of yoga and types of yoga. Examples of types of yoga are Raja, Tantra, and Hatha. _____ is the style referred to in this workbook.

2. Some styles are _____ and must not be taught unless the teacher is _____ from the school that owns the trademark. To do so would be unethical and illegal. If you teach in a way that pays homage to a certain style but you are not certified in that style, you should say you are teaching a class _____ that style. It's very important to be distinct about this because one is _____ intellectual property if one calls their class by a name that is protected by trademark.

Directions: Discuss the characteristics of each style, noting whether each is trademarked. Refer to the leaders guide or discussion with a teacher. Use a separate sheet of paper if you need more room.

Iyengar —

Bikram —

Anusara —

Ashtanga —

Power Yoga —

Gentle Yoga —

Restorative Yoga —

Yin Yoga —

Prenatal Yoga —

Children's Yoga —

Hot Yoga —

Y12SR —

Prime of Life Yoga —

Section 3: Limbs 1 and 2: Yamas and Niyamas

Ethics and Yoga

Name the Yama and Niyama that are the most meaningful to you and explain why.

Do you believe the Yamas and NiYamas are a good outline for assisting you in leading a more balanced and fulfilled life? Why or why not?

What does this mean to you? *"Its business, but it's never 'just business.'"* – Courtney Butler

Understanding and Being Your Authentic Self

Directions: Answer these questions, and feel free to continue on a separate sheet of paper, in the extra pages at the back of this book, or in a journal if you desire.

What are your hobbies and interests?

What tough experiences have shaped you?

What positive experiences shaped you?

Review the Yamas and NiYamas. Can you take a current decision you're facing and use those guidelines to help you make it? What do you think may happen when you release fear and have faith in this ancient practice?

(Return to these questions after the decision is made.) After the above practice, how did you feel? When acted upon, what was the outcome?

Why do you practice yoga?

What does yoga mean to you?

What are your strengths and good qualities?

What are the areas in life you struggle with?

If you want to teach, why?

Who are your supporters?

What do you see yourself doing in life? Feel free to be bold in your answers!

Who are your greatest influencers and what is it about them that you wish to emulate?

What is your learning style? (Auditory, Visual, Kinesthetic (Doing), Other)?

What do you think teaching will look like? If you want to own a studio, be a workshop leader, or own a school, discuss what that will look like and the steps you believe you need to follow to get there. If you don't want to teach, take a goal and break it down into the three steps necessary to reach it.

What is your expectation of the financial gain from teaching yoga? What is that expectation based upon?

Understanding the Student and Your Role as a Teacher

Yoga Teacher Interview: Find a yoga teacher who has been teaching at least five years (if available). Review their bio online (if available) beforehand, draft questions, and interview them. You might ask them how their yoga practice began and how they became a teacher. What were their expectations when they started? How does their reality differ from their expectations? What they have learned? Ask many questions and, if applicable, share with your teaching or book group.

Go to City-Data.com, Trulia, or another similar site to find out more about your community. Here are some questions for which you may already know the answers, or can find them with an easy internet search.

What is the population in your community and surrounding areas?

What ages are represented the most? Is it a young community, a retirement community, or both?

What types and styles of yoga are offered in the community? Where are they? How much do they cost? What are the teachers' backgrounds?

Is there a niche not being filled? Is there oversaturation in one area?

What are some barriers to teaching in this community? Consider things like oversaturation, cheap yoga, etc.

Questions for Teachers

Directions: Use the data and information you collected above to answer the questions below.

What does my community need?

What can I do to give back to my community?

What is my time worth versus what can people in my area afford to pay?

What are the demographics of my area? (Check City-Data.com.)

Observe with a critical eye the health clubs, yoga studios, and other similar venues you enter. What do you notice about the surroundings? What are the physical characteristics of their patrons? What are their patrons' personalities and preferences? What does their advertising and staff tell you about them? What can you learn by simply observing?

What is the population of students I expect to be serving or currently serve?

Do I have or perceive any special needs in my class/classes?

Am I comfortable teaching people who have physical abilities differing from me?

Am I willing to learn how to do hands-on assist and modifications in a safe way?

Do I consider a class in a holistic way (seeing the students as emotional and spiritual human beings as well as just physical bodies)?

Section 4: Physical and Energetic Anatomy

Physical Anatomy: Human Systems

Directions: Match the human system to its appropriate description.

- Circulatory (includes cardiovas-
  cular and lymphatic systems)
- Digestive
- Endocrine
- Integumentary
- Muscular
- Nervous
- Reproductive
- Respiratory
- Skeletal
- Special Sense
- Urinary

_____ bones, joints, cartilage, and connective tissue

_____ kidneys, ureters, bladder, and urethra

_____ skeletal, smooth, and cardiac muscles

_____ heart, blood vessels, blood and lymphatic system, lymphatic
vessels, and lymph

_____ mouth, pharynx, esophagus, stomach, small and large intestines,
accessory organs such as gallbladder and pancreas

_____ mouth, nasal cavity, bronchia, trachea, pharynx lungs and lobes, ribs

_____ brain, spinal cord, and all peripheral nerves

_____ eye, ear, nose, and taste buds

_____ glands and hormones produced by glands—pituitary, thyroid,
adrenal, thymus, pineal gland, pancreas, ovaries, and testes

_____ skin, hair, nails, glands

_____ sex organs

Directions: Use the words below to fill in the blanks.

- ball and socket
- calming
- cartilage
- collagen
- condyloid or ellipsoidal
- cortisol
- extend
- extends
- fascia
- gliding
- health
- hinge
- inhale
- joints
- ligaments
- massage
- pivot
- relaxation effect
- saddle
- skeletal
- tendons

1. The _____ system creates the framework for the body.

2. The six types of joints are:
   1.
   2.
   3.
   4.
   5.
   6.

3. _____ serves as the soft tissue that prevents our bones from clanking or rubbing together.

4. _____ is the body's most abundant protein and is the substance that holds the body together.

5. _____ connect muscle to bone.

6. _____ connect bone to bone.

7. _____ separates as well as connects everything in the body. It is like a stocking over the body holding everything together.

8. Synovial fluid has a _____ effect on the nervous system. It is found in the _____.

9. Muscles contract and _____.

10. Every time you contract a muscle, the opposite muscle _____.

11. In yoga, twists help to _____ the internal organs.

12. Some medical professionals believe that the _____, along with the blood flow to the belly and reproductive organs, can assist with fertility.

13. Yoga postures, breathing, and meditation reduce stress which in turn reduces the amount of _____ your body produces.

14. Yoga is helpful for respiratory conditions because it teaches the body to fully _____ and exhale, thus expanding lung capacity and the life and _____ of the lungs.

Energetic Anatomy

Directions: Use the words below to fill in the blanks.

- ama
- brain
- disease
- holistic
- integrative
- life
- oil rubbing
- spine
- 72,000

1. While Western medicine tends to deal with people on a gross anatomy level, Eastern medicine takes a more _____ approach.

2. With this understanding, we are seeing a rise in _____ medicine.

3. Ayurveda is often called the "Science of _____."

4. In Ayurveda, the cleansing practice of Panchakarma includes yoga, meditation, cleansing diet, pranayama, herbal tinctures, _____, and other specific treatments.

5. There are _____ Nadis. 108 are said to be of great importance.

6. A sticky substance that causes a blockage in the body is called a _____.

7. The 7 main Chakras line up with the _____, _____, and endocrine system.

Directions: Match the three most important nadis to their appropriate description.

- Ida
- Sushumna
- Pingala

_____ Left side of the body. Connects with the left nostril. Cool, light, airy, more yin quality. Controls mental processes.

_____ Right side of the body. Connects with right nostril. Dark, warm, heavy, more yang quality. Controls vital processes.

_____ The primary Nadi going up the spine, around which the other two primary nadis double helix. The pathway to heightened consciousness or spiritual awakening.

Directions: Match the koshas—the five facets of the human being according to ayurvedic science—to their appropriate description.

1. Annamayakosha
2. Pranamayakosha
3. Manomayakosha
4. Vijnyanamayakosha
5. Anadamayakosha

_____ The physical body. The form, solid structure, and balance of the body through all five elements: earth, water, fire, air, and space.

_____ The energetic body, including chakras and energy channels. The intake and flow of prana (life force) in the body.

_____ The psycho-emotional body. Drives emotional responses such as fight or flight. Blockages from stress can manifest into physical or mental illness.

_____ The wisdom body. Wisdom, intuition, insight, the witness observer that recognizes life patterns and how to change them.

_____ The bliss body. The true self is one of inner contentment and connection to the divine or that of a greater understanding than what is tangible on this earth.

Elements

Directions: List the five elements that make up the doshas.

1.

2.

3.

4.

5.

Doshas

Directions: Match the dosha to its description.

- Pitta
- Kapha
- Vata

_____ Combines air and space. Person tends to be light in structure, typically taller, or petite and thinner. Subtle, creative, and full of new ideas.

_____ Mostly fire with some water. Person tends towards medium builds and are more muscular. Generally friendly, outgoing, strong, brave.

_____ Combines earth and water. Reminiscent of turtles, they are heavier in build and have larger frames. They move more slowly and are gentle in nature.

The Chakras

Directions: Use the words below to fill in the blanks.

- energy
- one hundred fourteen
- ROYGBIV
- seven
- wheel

1. Chakra means _____.

2. The Chakras are _____ centers in the body.

3. Most are familiar with _____ main chakras that line up from the base of the pelvic floor to the top of the head, but in total, there are _____ chakras.

4. The acronym you can use to help you remember the colors of the chakras and their order is _____.

Fill in the charts using the Guide, working with a teacher, or using your own tools to research.

First Chakra

Location:	Affirmation:
Element:	Shadow Emotions:
Color:	Impacts:
Function:	Postures:
Verb:	Kosha:

Second Chakra

Location:

Element:

Color:

Function:

Verb:

Affirmation:

Shadow Emotions:

Impacts:

Postures:

Kosha:

Third Chakra

Location:

Element:

Color:

Function:

Verb:

Affirmation:

Shadow Emotions:

Impacts:

Postures:

Kosha:

Fourth Chakra

Location:

Element:

Color:

Function:

Verb:

Affirmation:

Shadow Emotions:

Impacts:

Postures:

Kosha:

Firth Chakra

Location:

Element:

Color:

Function:

Verb:

Affirmation:

Shadow Emotions:

Impacts:

Postures:

Kosha:

Sixth Chakra

Location: Affirmation:

Element: Shadow Emotions:

Color: Impacts:

Function: Postures:

Verb: Kosha:

Seventh Chakra

Location: Affirmation:

Element: Shadow Emotions:

Color: Impacts:

Function: Postures:

Verb: Kosha:

Mantras, Mudras, and Bandhas

Directions: Match these ancient healing arts with their descriptions.
- Mantras
- Mudras
- Bandhas

_____ Hymns or words repeated to bring higher consciousness and awareness, much the same way as an affirmation. Certain ones are associated with certain chakras.

_____ Hand gestures that are said to influence the flow of energy in the body.

_____ Locks that are used to control energy in the body.

Four Types of Bandhas

Directions: Match the proper bandha with its description.

- Mula
- Uddiyana
- Maha

- Jalandhara

_____ Bandha — locking of the pelvic floor, much like a Kegal, as if stopping the flow of urine.

_____ Bandha — Lifting of the diaphragm as if lifting the muscles used when vomiting. Teaching oneself to hold this bandha while exhaling and inhaling often takes many years of practice and so is uncommon hatha yoga classes.

_____ Bandha — There are two forms of this chin lock. One is to take the chin and rest it in the soft spot in the low neck below the thyroid. The other (and the easier) is to hold the head erect over the torso, put a flat hand up to the nose and push back one inch, slightly lowering the chin.

_____ Bandha — When all three bandhas are done at once.

- Hand
- Foot

Hasta Bandha — "_____ Lock"
Pada Bandha — "_____ Lock"

Movement and Balance of Energetic Anatomy

Directions: Use the words below to fill in the blanks.

- asana
- meditation
- pranayama
- six

A balanced practice should always include moving the spine in all _____ directions as well as including _____, _____, and _____.

Section 5: Limbs 3 and 4: Pranayama and Asana

Pranayama

Directions: Use the words below to fill in the blanks. Note that oxygen and pranayama will each be used twice.

- carbon dioxide
- energy
- heart
- intercostals
- oxygen

- parasympathetic
- prana
- pranayama
- spine

1. _____ means "life force."

2. _____ is the movement of not just oxygen, but _____ in the body. When we breathe in _____, we are bringing a life-giving substance into our body that we must have to live. When we exhale _____, we are expelling what we don't need or what is toxic to our body. Without each process, we would die. When we exhale, plants and trees turn our carbon dioxide into _____, which is returned to us. Without them we would not survive. This furthers our connection or oneness with the world.

3. Pranayama massages the _____. The _____ is lengthened, the _____ are stretched, and the lungs are exercised all with the expansion and contraction of breath. Simultaneously, the nervous system is bought under control with properly practiced pranayama the body goes into a . . .

4. _____ state, relaxing and renewing the body mind.

5. When beginning a yoga practice, it is best to stick to the basics of _____.

In your own words, define the four basic types of pranayama practice most often taught in general hatha yoga classes.

Basic Belly Breathing or Two-Part Breath —

Durga or Three-Part Breath —

Ujjayi or Victory Breath —

Nodi Shodhana or Alternate Nostril Breath —

Safety Symbol:
What conditions might require students to take precautions in their pranayama practice? What should students do if they aren't feeling well while practicing? What is the safest method of pranayama for high-risk students or groups?

Asana

Directions: Use the words below to fill in the blanks. Some of the words will be used twice.

- balance
- beginning
- bell curve
- contraindications
- glaucoma
- high blood pressure

- inversions
- middle
- modifications
- physical
- position
- pregnancy

- props
- seat
- shavasana
- six
- sukhasana
- vinyasa

1. Today, asana is commonly used to refer to a practitioner's _____. The word's literal translation is to take an easy, comfortable _____. The oldest known pose documented in writing is easy pose or _____.

2. There are some elements to Hatha yoga that lend a class to have overall _____.

3. Make sure the spine is being moved in all_____ directions. This ensures _____ and energetic balance in the body. Add safe _____ where appropriate for you or your students.

4. The class should have a _____, _____, and an end. Follow a _____ method. There will be a warm up to prepare the body, a core that focuses on the style and type of class you are practicing or teaching, and a cool down with _____ and meditation.

5. _____ is generally considered to mean linking postures with breath.

6. _____ can be used to modify poses, lengthen the arms and legs, to make postures more comfortable, or to deepen a pose. In restorative yoga, these are used to hold poses and support the body, and in yin yoga they are used to make postures more accessible.

7. Before teaching a class with advanced poses, teachers should be trained by someone who is very safety-oriented, and have extensive knowledge of _____, _____, and _____. Always remember that a pose done in a few minutes can cause an injury that is lifelong.

8. Before beginning a class what are at least three of the major health concerns you should be asking about? Feel free to add others to this list.

   1.

   2.

   3.

Asana Modifications

Safety Symbol:
List several instances in which modifications of poses should be given. Give examples of two modifications with the names of the poses, the reasons for the modifications, and detailed explanations of the modifications.

Asanas/Poses

In the coming pages, use the Guide to assist you in filling out the chart for each pose. If you need more space, use the extra pages at the back of this book or additional sheets of paper.

1. **Easy Seated**

    Sanskrit:

    Type of Pose:

    Benefits:

    Chakras:

    Verbal Cues:

    Lines of Energy:

    Contraindications:

    Modifications and Suggested Props:

    Assist or Adjustments:

    Variations:

    Stick Figure or Detailed Description:

2. **Staff**

    Sanskrit:

    Type of Pose:

    Benefits:

    Chakras:

    Verbal Cues:

Lines of Energy:

Contraindications:

Modifications and Suggested Props:

Assist or Adjustments:

Variations:

Stick Figure or Detailed Description:

3. **Cobbler**

Sanskrit:

Type of Pose:
Benefits:

Chakras:

Verbal Cues:

Lines of Energy:

Contraindications:

Modifications and Suggested Props:

Assist or Adjustments:

Variations:

Stick Figure or Detailed Description:

4. Lateral Side Lean

Sanskrit:

Type of Pose:

Benefits:

Chakras:

Verbal Cues:

Lines of Energy:

Contraindications:

Modifications and Suggested Props:

Assist or Adjustments:

Variations:

Stick Figure or Detailed Description:

5. **Seated Spinal Twist**

Sanskrit:

Type of Pose:

Benefits:

Chakras:

Verbal Cues:

Lines of Energy:

Contraindications:

Modifications and Suggested Props:

Assist or Adjustments:

Variations:

Stick Figure or Detailed Description:

6. **Cat – Cow**

Sanskrit:

Type of Pose:

Benefits:

Chakras:

Verbal Cues:

Lines of Energy:

Contraindications:

Modifications and Suggested Props:

Assist or Adjustments:

Variations:

Stick Figure or Detailed Description:

7. **Child's Pose**

Sanskrit:

Type of Pose:

Benefits:

Chakras:

Verbal Cues:

Lines of Energy:

Contraindications:

Modifications and Suggested Props:

Assist or Adjustments:

Variations:

Stick Figure or Detailed Description:

8. **Downward Facing Dog (Down Dog)**

Sanskrit:

Type of Pose:

Benefits:

Chakras:

Verbal Cues:

Lines of Energy:

Contraindications:

Modifications and Suggested Props:

Assist or Adjustments:

Variations:

Stick Figure or Detailed Description:

9. **Standing Forward Fold**

Sanskrit:

Type of Pose:

Benefits:

Chakras:

Verbal Cues:

Lines of Energy:

Contraindications:

Modifications and Suggested Props:

Assist or Adjustments:

Variations:

Stick Figure or Detailed Description:

10. **Mountain**

Sanskrit:

Type of Pose:

Benefits:

Chakras:

Verbal Cues:

Lines of Energy:

Contraindications:

Modifications and Suggested Props:

Assist or Adjustments:

Variations:

Stick Figure or Detailed Description:

11. Warrior 1

Sanskrit:

Type of Pose:

Benefits:

Chakras:

Verbal Cues:

Lines of Energy:

Contraindications:

Modifications and Suggested Props:

Assist or Adjustments:

Variations:

Stick Figure or Detailed Description:

12. Warrior 2

Sanskrit:

Type of Pose:

Benefits:

Chakras:

Verbal Cues:

Lines of Energy:

Contraindications:

Modifications and Suggested Props:

Assist or Adjustments:

Variations:

Stick Figure or Detailed Description:

13. Triangle

Sanskrit:

Type of Pose:

Benefits:

Chakras:

Verbal Cues:

Lines of Energy:

Contraindications:

Modifications and Suggested Props:

Assist or Adjustments:

Variations:

Stick Figure or Detailed Description:

14. Pyramid

Sanskrit:

Type of Pose:

Benefits:

Chakras:

Verbal Cues:

Lines of Energy:

Contraindications:

Modifications and Suggested Props:

Assist or Adjustments:

Variations:

Stick Figure or Detailed Description:

15. Wide-Legged Forward Fold

Sanskrit:

Type of Pose:

Benefits:

Chakras:

Verbal Cues:

Lines of Energy:

Contraindications:

Modifications and Suggested Props:

Assist or Adjustments:

Variations:

Stick Figure or Detailed Description:

16. Chair

Sanskrit:

Type of Pose:

Benefits:

Chakras:

Verbal Cues:

Lines of Energy:

Contraindications:

Modifications and Suggested Props:

Assist or Adjustments:

Variations:

Stick Figure or Detailed Description:

17. Tree

Sanskrit:

Type of Pose:

Benefits:

Chakras:

Verbal Cues:

Lines of Energy:

Contraindications:

Modifications and Suggested Props:

Assist or Adjustments:

Variations:

Stick Figure or Detailed Description:

18. Locust

Sanskrit:

Type of Pose:

Benefits:

Chakras:

Verbal Cues:

Lines of Energy:

Contraindications:

Modifications and Suggested Props:

Assist or Adjustments:

Variations:

Stick Figure or Detailed Description:

19. Cobra and Sphinx

Sanskrit:

Type of Pose:

Benefits:

Chakras:

Verbal Cues:

Lines of Energy:

Contraindications:

Modifications and Suggested Props:

Assist or Adjustments:

Variations:

Stick Figure or Detailed Description:

20. Seated Forward Bend and Half-Seated Forward Bend

Sanskrit:

Type of Pose:

Benefits:

Chakras:

Verbal Cues:

Lines of Energy:

Contraindications:

Modifications and Suggested Props:

Assist or Adjustments:

Variations:

Stick Figure or Detailed Description:

21. Shoulder Stand

Sanskrit:

Type of Pose:

Benefits:

Chakras:

Verbal Cues:

Lines of Energy:

Contraindications:

Modifications and Suggested Props:

Assist or Adjustments:

Variations:

Stick Figure or Detailed Description:

22. Bridge

Sanskrit:

Type of Pose:

Benefits:

Chakras:

Verbal Cues:

Lines of Energy:

Contraindications:

Modifications and Suggested Props:

Assist or Adjustments:

Variations:

Stick Figure or Detailed Description:

23. Reclined Spinal Twist

Sanskrit:

Type of Pose:

Benefits:

Chakras:

Verbal Cues:

Lines of Energy:

Contraindications:

Modifications and Suggested Props:

Assist or Adjustments:

Variations:

Stick Figure or Detailed Description:

24. Knees to Chest

Sanskrit:

Type of Pose:

Benefits:

Chakras:

Verbal Cues:

Lines of Energy:

Contraindications:

Modifications and Suggested Props:

Assist or Adjustments:

Variations:

Stick Figure or Detailed Description:

25. Corpse

Sanskrit:

Type of Pose:

Benefits:

Chakras:

Verbal Cues:

Lines of Energy:

Contraindications:

Modifications and Suggested Props:

Assist or Adjustments:

Variations:

Stick Figure or Detailed Description:

Section 6: Limbs 5 through 8

In your own words, describe limbs 5 through 8 as you understand them, or as you would explain them to someone else. If you have experienced each of these limbs yourself, go into detail about your own experience.

Limb 5 — Pratyahara

Limb 6 — Dharana

Limb 7 — Dhyana

Limb 8 — Samadhi

Meditation

Name 3 ways you can teach meditation, and give a brief description of each approach.

1.

2.

3.

Share three resources you can use for more information on meditation

    1.

    2.

    3.

From what you have studied and learned in *The Mud & The Lotus: A Guide for Students of Yoga*, from your teachers, or in your own research or experience, what would be one way to help someone become more grounded when they feel that life is spinning out of control?

Section 7: Yoga Business Basics

Finding Work and Getting Paid

Directions: Use the words below to fill in the blanks.

- style
- sub
- try out
- vary
- work

The amount a yoga teacher makes will _____ depending on where and what they are teaching, and who they are working for. When you first start out it's best to take classes in the places you would like to _____. Yoga styles vary greatly so you may find that you like one _____ or vibe better than another. Then ask the teacher, administrator, or owner if you could be on the _____ list. They may ask you to _____ so they can experience the way you teach.

Name 4 places yoga is or could be offered:
1.
2.
3.
4.

What is the difference between being a contractor and an employee?

How can you find out what you should be getting paid to teach yoga?

Name as many expenses as you can that a brick and mortar studio would incur?

How can you determine what you should charge for:

Yoga classes?

Private classes?

Intensives?

You would like to offer yoga to those who may not be able to afford your classes. How can you achieve this without going out of business?

You would like to rent space from a local dance studio or church. What's the average percentage you'll expect to earn for doing something like this?

If you don't pay a percentage, how will you know what the rent will be?

How can you figure out if renting space or paying a percentage will be worth it? How will you figure how many students you need on average to cover cost? List all the costs that you might incur.

What is the difference between a workshop and an intensive?

What should your credentials be to offer workshops for Continuing Education requirements with Yoga Alliance?

What is a yoga party and what population would it address?

What is corporate yoga and what is the current going rate?

One will generally have a few years' experience and be an ERYT before offering workshops. If you are not an ERYT, you might offer intensives until you have those credentials. Answer these questions to assist you in understanding associated costs and profits.

What percentage does a workshop host keep?

What percentage does the presenter keep?

What expenses are associated with hosting a workshop?

Are the expenses deducted before or after the host and presenter are paid?

Looking at Yourself as a Teacher

Teaching can be exhausting if you find yourself caring too much for others and not caring for yourself in return. Review your desires, needs, and expectations before embarking on this journey. Here are some questions to ask/explore:

What times of the day and what days of the week are best for me and/or my family/those close to me?

Are there certain times of the year when I'm able to work more? Should I sub, do I want to teach full time, or both?

How many classes do I feel like I can reasonably handle and not take away from my own practice, family, loved ones, etc.?

How much do I need to make per month teaching yoga?

What kind of teaching do I enjoy? Private yoga, classes, intensives, corporate yoga, working the retail desk at a yoga studio, administration of a yoga program, or something else?

What type of atmosphere works best for me? Do I like a gym setting where I can also work out? Do I like the feel of a studio and being with other serious yogis? Do I like a power yoga studio, a gentle style studio, or one that offers many types of yoga? Do I want to work in a studio that caters to younger people, older people, middle-aged people, or a mix?

Business Ethics

Directions: Use the words below to fill in the blanks.

- competing
- hurt

Teaching for two or more _____ businesses may be bad business, unethical, and may _____ your relationship with owners and administrators. If you choose to go work somewhere else, it is always best to communicate with your current employer or the owner of the studio before moving forward to avoid miscommunication.

You are working at a studio and need to earn more money but don't want work for a competing studio. What are some things you could do to earn more money in the field of yoga?

How can you ethically teach yoga in a variety of places without causing problems with the people you work for?

Advertising and Marketing Ethically

In order for potential students to know about you, you must get the message out. Here are some questions to ask yourself before you begin marketing yourself.

Who are you as a teacher (credentials & experience)?

What is the day and time you are offering your class or event?

What is the cost?

Where is the location?

What is the style or type of yoga offered / class description?

What message do you want to send (what is the need you are filling and how do you want the students to feel about the class)?

What is your budget ?

Are you working solo or in conjunction with a host? What are his/her responsibilities and what are your responsibilities?

Mock Flier Assignment: Make a mock flier for your class you are offering, use a sheet of paper to draw in the words and pictures, use cut outs from a magazine, or you can do something separately on the computer.

Marketing Budgets

When you have no money in your budget, what are three ways to get the word out about your class?

If you have $150 in your budget and one month before your class, what are two ways to get the word out?

If you have $300 or more in your monthly budget for marketing, what are two ways to get the word out?

What should you consider when choosing a location for your yoga classes or studio?

Lifestyles of Health and Sustainability (LOHAS) Markets

Though we may not like to put people in boxes, with regard to marketing, it is important to think in terms of what groups of people are spending or might spend their money on. This allows you to effectively use your dollars and energy to connect with students and customers who are looking for someone like you. For advertising purposes, answering these questions will help, as well as observing and documenting what works or doesn't work for other similar businesses, and/or simply looking online for ideas.
We know the market for yoga is generally the "LOHAS" market Explain in your own words what this acronym means and your potential target audience (e.g. where do they live and shop, what do they buy, and what are their habits).

How do you know if your marketing is working?

Websites and Social Media

When creating a website or social media account for your business, what basic information needs to be available?

Ethics in the Yoga World

What is the golden rule?

Do you trust that if you live by the tenets of yoga that you can be a successful yoga teacher?

Everyone's yoga path is different. It's great to learn from and even follow people you admire, however we all need to teach from an authentic core of who we are and what we enjoy and want to share—this is our unique gift to the world and will not be the same as anyone else's. Years of teaching, showing up, being kind, being ethical, recognizing what you are good at and not focusing on trying to be like others is the path to true authenticity as a yoga teacher. Not everyone will be attracted to your style of teaching, but others might love your style. This is how you build and keep clientele.

As you build clientele:

Is it ever okay to use someone else's contact list for your own resources without their permission?

You have worked for a local gym for three years and you are leaving to start your own studio. You know it's not ethical to contact the students from the studio. How do you go about reaching people and letting them know where you are going?

Mini Business Plan

Directions: Look over all the information you have gathered and answer the questions below to the best of your ability.

Do you want to teach or simply study and advance your knowledge of yoga?

How often would you like to teach?

What style of yoga would you like to teach?

Where would you like to teach?

What is the best schedule for you?

How much do you expect to make?

Connect the work you want to do with anticipate income. For instance – 2 classes per week at $30 each and 1 private lesson for $50 would equal $110 a week/ approximately $440 a month. What is your expected weekly/monthly income for the work you want to do?

Will you have any expenses or overhead? If so, list all costs you may incur.

How will you market your classes?

Do you know what your market is?

What will you charge?

How will you avoid burnout?

What income do you need to live monthly? Can you afford to work at yoga full time or part time?

Section 8: The Yoga Lifestyle

What does a yoga lifestyle mean to you?

Has its meaning changed for you from the first time you took a class until now? If so, how?

Living Your Yoga

While yoga itself isn't goal-oriented, you can use the tools and guidelines yoga offers to lead a content and fulfilling life. Below, I share an approach to help you with your own life goals that I use in my role as a Certified Yoga Therapist and Certified Solution Focused Coach as I work with clients. When we pair the somatic (related to the body, e.g. the asanas) and the cognitive practices (meditation, workbook, discussions, thinking, and writing), we begin to change old patterns and habits. You may find as you embark on the next phase of your yoga journey that tying together this practice with yoga is beneficial to help you actualize the many thoughts on ideas that may be swirling in your mind as you complete this training.

What are your goals for one month, six months, one year, three years, and ten years? You may list personal and work or you can choose one. (Choose one to do the first study, but after that, you can apply this approach to any area of your life.) An example "Saving $1,000" is provided below.

On a scale of one to ten, ten being the goal is met, how close are you to achieving each of your goals?

What are your obstacles in achieving these goals?

In the past what is the closest you have come to achieving your goal?

Who are your supporters?

Now let's break down your goal and give it a timeline.

First choose a short-term goal that can be achieved in one month. Then use this application for long-term goals as well.

Name the goal:

What is the timeline to reach the goal?

Why do you want to achieve this? How will you feel if you do achieve this?

How is this goal "yoga"? You are achieving your goals by using the methods of visualization, affirmation, and positive thinking. Through asana, pranayama, and meditation you are strengthening your sources (body and mind) to keep you from getting emotionally and physically exhausted which in turn helps you stay motivated and encouraged to have a balanced life. When we mix movement and mental awareness together we begin to change samskaras (pathways) or neural pathways in the body and mind.

Who are your supporters? What is your plan for reaching out when you need support?

What are your obstacles?

What is your plan for dealing with obstacles?

What is the first thing you need to do to get started?

What is the second step you'll need to take?

What is the third?

First Example: Save $1000 for Emergency Fund

(Remember, this is just an example. Goals should be achievable. If you only make $1000 a month, your goal may be much less.)

1. Do a daily balanced asana practice 3 x per week. Include simple pranayama to keep my mind and body balanced and helps me achieve any goal.

2. Prepare an affirmation in the present positive tense: "I have $1000 in savings."

3. Daily, say my affirmation and visualize my goal, completed. Visualize the steps I must take each day and week.

4. Keep a copy of my notes nearby and review.

5. Do the task that leads you closer to your goal.

6. Meditate daily and use guided meditations in line with my goal.

1st Ten Days: Save $375

- Have a garage sale
- Open a savings account with the money
- Put 10% of my paycheck in the account
- Take at least twenty items to the resale shop

2nd Ten Days: Save Another $375

- Sell some of my things on Facebook Big Furniture for Sale
- Do some extra work. For me it may be offering a yoga intensive.
- Spend less, eat out less. Save the money I would spend on other things. Three meals out a week would be $60. Eat at home and put that $60 in the bank.
- Put 10% of paycheck in bank

3rd Ten Days: Save the Balance of $250

- On day 30, see if I have any money at resale shop
- Get creative and find something else to sell, maybe some old gold jewelry I don't need.
- Continue to identify needs versus wants and save the money I would have spent on wants, even $10 at a time. Watch movies at home and save. Take a walk instead of shop.
- Put 10% of paycheck in the bank.

Second Example: Lose 5% of Body Weight to Improve Health

I want to lose 10lbs because I have some health conditions and the doctors say if I can lose 5% of my body weight my health should improve. I will feel healthier and happier if I achieve this. My obstacles are eating out with friends and family, being too tired to cook, not having the proper foods in the house, not having enough time to exercise. My supporter is my fiancé who is a healthy eater and works out.

1. Take supplements to support blood sugar and hormones.

2. Grocery shop for healthy foods that support my diet.

3. Walk ½ mile three times a week and do 15 minutes of yoga with 5 minute meditation.

4. Do a single hour-long yoga class and walk one mile, once during the week.

5. Drink water, no sweetened drinks of foods, avoid fried foods and processed foods, and eat at home as much as possible or pack food.

6. Check in with my girlfriend, Sarah, to whom I feel accountable.

    1st Ten Days: Lose 3.5 lbs (from 149 to 145.5)

    - Repeat steps 1–5

    2nd Ten Days: Lose 3.5 lbs (from 145.5 to 142)

    - Repeat steps 1–5
    - Add: Increase to two yoga classes per week for one hour and two days a week walking a mile, add two days of strength training.

    3rd Ten Days: Check in and see where I am, hopefully I am at 142 and have 3 lbs to go to reach my goal of 139.

    - Repeat all steps. If it's going well I will continue with all steps as they are previously.
    - I'll call my supporters or coach and get support. I know the last three lbs will be tough.
    - If I'm not losing as much as I was I'll need to evaluate my diet, portions, and exercise.

    30 day check in: I am hopefully now down to 139 and want to maintain my weight. I'll continue with things as they are and watch myself each month. If I gain weight I'll get right back on track and get it off as soon as possible.

Living a Happy Life with Yoga

Make a list of things that make you happy. Make a list of things you can let go of that are not serving you. Keep these lists nearby, review at them, revise them, and practice the contents of your lists often.

What makes me happy? (Example: *Taking my dog for a walk.*)

What can I let go of or what is not serving me? (Example: *Watching two hours of TV per day.*)

Section 9: Sample Classes and Guidelines

How and why might Namaste, Shanti, and/or Om be used or combined to bring class to a close?

Describe with your words and draw in stick figures a one hour class from beginning to end. Include details about how you would open and close (intention & meditation). You may not include all the postures I have in the book or in Section 9, however your class should flow and create balance.

Workbook Key

The following key is for fill-in-the-blanks and matching sections only.

Section 1

What is Yoga

1. yoke, unite
2. yuj, bind
3. yogis, yogini, yogi

A Brief and Basic History of Yoga

1. Lifestyle
2. Debate
3. The Vedic Period, Vedas, Veda
4. Pre-classical Yoga
5. Classical Period
6. Post Classical Period
7. Modern Period

1. Upanishads
2. Bhagavad Gita
3. Sutras
4. Hatha Yoga Pradapika

Section 2

Credentialing

1. require
2. not
3. licensed

Yoga Alliance

1. credentialing
2. nonprofit
3. certificate

Schools

1. 200RYS
2. 300RYS
3. 500RYS
4. RCYS
5. RPYS
6. YACEP

Teachers

1. RYT 200
2. ERYT 200
3. RYT 500
4. ERYT 500
5. RPYT
6. RCYT

Structuring a Class

1. Bell Curve, beginning, middle, end
2. (1) forward bending (2) backward bending (3/4) lateral left/right (5/6) twist left/right
3. forward bends and twists
4. backbends and twists
5. body, mind

1. introduce
2. props
3. medical conditions
4. at home
5. heart, twist, inversions

Styles of Yoga

1. Hatha
2. trademarked, certified, inspired, stealing

Section 3

Human Systems

- Skeletal
- Urinary
- Muscular
- Circulatory
- Digestive
- Respiratory
- Nervous
- Special Senses
- Endocrine
- Integumentary
- Reproductive

1. skeletal
2. (1) gliding (2) hinge (3) saddle (4) condyloid or ellipsoidal (5) ball and socket (6) pivot
3. cartilage
4. collagen
5. tendons
6. ligaments
7. fascia
8. calming, joints
9. extend
10. extends
11. massage
12. relaxation effect
13. cortisol
14. inhale, health

Section 4

Energetic Anatomy
1. holistic
2. integrative
3. life
4. oil rubbing
5. 72,000
6. ama
7. spine, brain

Nadis
- Ida
- Pingala
- Sushumna

Koshas
1,2,3,4,5

Elements
1. Earth
2. Water
3. Fire
4. Air
5. Space

Doshas
- Vata
- Kapha
- Pitta

Chakras
1. wheel
2. energy
3. seven, one hundred fourteen
4. ROYGBIV

Mudra, Mantra and Bandha
- Mantra
- Mudra
- Banda

Bandhas
- Mula
- Uddiyana
- Maha
- Jalahandra
- Hand
- Foot

Hand and Foot Lock
1. Hasta
2. Pada

200

Section 5

Pranayama
1. lifeforce
2. pranayama, energy, oxygen, carbon dioxide, oxygen
3. heart, spine, intercostals
4. parasympathetic
5. pranayama

Asana
1. posture, seat, sukhasana
2. balance
3. six, physical, modifications
4. beginning, middle, bell curve, shavasana
5. vinyasa
6. props
7. props, modifications, contratindications
8. glaucoma, high blood pressure, and pregnancy

Section 7

Finding Work and Getting Paid

vary, work, style, sub, try out

Business Ethics

competing, hurt

Index

About the Author, 211

Adjusting and Assisting, 31

Acknowledgements, 198

Advertising and Marketing Ethically, 109

Ahimsa — Non-violence, 22

Ama, 41

An Approach from Early Childhood
  Education, 40

Anusara, 17

Aparigraha — Non-attachment, 22

Asana, 2, 3, 4, 38, 53-54

Ashtanga, 17

Asteya — No Stealing, 22

Ayurveda, 40

Bandhas, 47, 48, 82, 83

Baptiste, Baron, 7

Basics of Energetic Anatomy, 49

Bell, Baxter, 7

Bhakti, 3, 136

Bikram, 17

Biobliography, 127-129

Birch, Bereyl Bender, 8

Brahmacharya — Moderation, 22

Business Ethics in the Yoga World, 113

Chakras, The, 44, 45, 47, 49, 61-88

Children's Yoga, 17

Choudhury, Bikram, 8

Circulatory System, 34

Clark, Bernie, 8

Class Beginning, 13

Class End, 15

Class Middle, 14

Classical Period, 6

Corn, Seane, 8

Credentialing, 11

Desikachar, 7

Determining Per Class Charge, 103

Dharana, 2, 89, 91, 177

Dhyana, 89, 92, 177

Digestive System, 34

Doshas, 42, 43, 46, 152

E-RYT 200, 12

E-RYT 500, 12

Eight Limbs of Yoga, The, 1-2, 21, 51, 89, 133

Endocrine System, 33, 34, 146

Energetic Anatomy, 39-40, 49

Energy Anatomy Chart, 46

Ethics and Yoga, 21

Expectations of Practice and Teaching, 27

Finding Work and Getting Paid, 97

Five Points of Yoga, The 3

Folan, Lilias, 8, 91

For Studio owners, Prospective Owners, and
  Teachers, 99

Forest, Anna, 8

Friend, John, 8

Full Sun Salutation, 58

Gannon, Sharon, 8

Gates, Rolf, 8

Gaze or Drishti, 56

Gentle Yoga, 17

Gunas, 49

Gyms and Colleges, 98

Half Sun Salutation, 58

Hands-on Adjustments, 31, 61-88

Hatha, 3, 16-18, 53

Hot Yoga, 17

Identifying Community Needs, 31

Income Sources for Yoga Teachers, 103

Integumentary System, 34

International Association of Yoga Therapists
  (IAYT), 12

Ishvara Pranidhana — Surrendering to a
  Higher Power, 23

Iyengar, 17

Iyengar, B.K.S., 7

Jnana, 3

Jois, K. Pattabhi, 7

Karma, 3

Kepner, John, 8

Koshas, 42, 44-46, 152
Kraftsow, Gary, 8
Krishnamacharya, Sri T., iii, 7
Lasiter, Judith Hanson, 8
Learning Styles, 30
Letter to Readers, i
Life, David, 8
Limb 1 — Yamas, 1, 21, 114, 117, 133, 145
Limb 2 — Niyamas, 2, 21, 114, 117, 133, 145
Limb 3 — Asana, 2, 53, 134
Limb 4 — Pranayama, 2, 51
Limb 5 — Pratyahara, 2, 89, 90
Limb 6 — Dharana, 2, 91
Limb 7 — Dhyana, 2, 89, 92, 177
Limb 8 — Samadhi, 2, 95
Limb, 8 limbs of Yoga, 1, 133, 134
Limbs 1 and 2: Yamas and Niyamas, 21
Limbs 3 and 4: Pranayama and Asana, 51
Limbs 5 through 8, 90
Living a Happy Life with Yoga, 118
Mantra, 3, 47
Mantras, Mudras, and Bandhas, 47
Marketing Budgets, 111
Meditation in Practice, 95
Modern Day Western Teachers, 7
Mohan, A.G., 7
Mudras, 47
Muscular System, 35, 36
Music, 18
My Lineage, iii
Myers, Nikki, 8
Nadis, 4, 41, 51
Nervous System, 36
Niyamas, 2, 21, 22
Niyamas, Ishvara Pranidhana - Surrender, 22
Niyamas, Santosha - Contentment, 2, 22, 133
Niyamas, Saucha - Cleanliness, 2, 22, 133
Niyamas, Svadhyaya- Spiritual Study, 2, 23, 134
Niyamas, Tapas - Discipline or Practice 2, 22, 134
Overview, 1

Payne, Larry, 8, 54
Permission Language, 16
Physical Anatomy/Systems of the Human Body, 33
Physical and Energetic Anatomy, 33
Poses, The, 56–88
  Bridge — Setu Bandhasana, 83
  Cat–Cow — Durga–Go, 66
  Chair — Utkatasana, 77
  Child's Pose — Balasana, 67
  Cobbler — Baddha Konasana, 63
  Cobra and Sphinx — Bhujangasana, 80
  Corpse — Shavasana, 87
  Down Dog — Adho Mukha Svanasana, 68
  Easy Seated Pose — Sukhasana, 61
  Knees to Chest — Apanasana, 86
  Lateral Side Leans — Ardha Parighasana, 64
  Locust — Shalabhasana, 79
  Mountain — Tadasana, 71
  Pyramid — Parsvottanasana, 75
  Reclined Spinal Twist Series — Jathara Parivartanasana, 84
  Seated Forward Bend and Half Seated Forward Bend — Paschimottanasana, 81
  Seated Spinal Twist — Paravritta Sukhasana, 65
  Shoulder Stand and Half Shoulder Stand — Sarvangasana and Viparita Karani, 82
  Staff — Dandasana, 62
  Standing Forward Fold — Uttanasana, 70
  Triangle — Trikonasana, 74
  Tree — Vrkshasana, 78
  Warrior 1 — Vira 1, 72
  Warrior 2 — Vira 2, 73
  Wide-Legged Forward Fold — Prasarita Padottanasana, 76
Positive Thinking and Meditation, 3
Post-Classical Period, 6
Power Yoga, 17
Practice of Teaching, The 11
Pranayama, 2, 51, 157
Pratyahara, 2, 90

Pre-Classical Period, 5
Preface, i
Prenatal Yoga, 17
Prime of Life Yoga, 18
Private Lessons, Intensives (Events), Parties, and Corporate Yoga, 107
Proper Breathing, 3
Proper Diet, 3
Proper Exercise, 3
Proper Relaxation, 3
Props, 54, 55
Raja, 3
RCYS, 11
RCYT, 12
Reproductive System, 36
Respiratory System, 37
Restorative Yoga, 18
RPYS, 12
RPYT, 12
RYS 200, 11
RYS 300, 11
RYS 500, 11
RYT 200, 12
RYT 500, 12
Samadhi, 2, 95
Sample Class, 121–125
Sample Class and Guideline, 121
Sample Joint-Opening Poses, 14
Sample Seated Meditation, 14
Samskaras, 42
Santosha — Contentment, 2, 23
Satya — Truthfulness, 1, 22
Saucha — Cleanliness, 2, 22
Shiffman, Erich, 8
Shiva Rea, 8
Skeletal System, 37, 38
Special Sense System, 39
State Licenses, 11
Staying in Business, 99
Structuring a Class: The Bell Curve Method, 13
Stryker, Rod, 9

Studio Location, 113
Studios, 98
Styles of Hatha Yoga, 16-17
Summing up Financials and Where to Teach, 109
Sun Salutation, 14, 58, 121, 122
Svadhyaya — Spiritual Study, 2, 23
Swami Satchidananda, 7
Tantra, 3
Tapas — Discipline or Practice, 2, 23
The Yoga Lifestyle, 117
Trademarked Yoga Styles, 17-18
Types of Yoga, 2
Understanding and Being Your Authentic Self, 24
Understanding the Student, 28
Urinary System, 39
Vedic Period, The, 5, 135
Verbal Cuing, 31, 61-88
Walden, Patricia, 9
Walking the Room for Safety, 30
What is Yoga?, 1
Working with Other Businesses: The Percentage Approach, 105
Y12SR, 18
YACEP, 12
Yamas, 1, 21
  Yamas, Ahimsa – Nonviolence, 1, 21, 133
  Yamas, Aparigraha – Nonattachment, 1, 21, 133
  Yamas, Asteya – Non-stealing, 1, 21, 133
  Yamas, Brahmacharya – Moderation, 1, 21, 133
  Yamas, Satya – Truthfulness, 1, 21, 133
Yee, Rodney, 9
Yin Yoga, 18
Yoga Alliance Credentialing, 11
Yoga Alliance School Designations, 11
Yoga Alliance Teacher Designations, 12
Yoga Business Basics, 97
Yoga Masters of India, 6
Yogananda, Paramahansa, 7

Acknowledgements

I am not sure there is a way to thank everyone who has taught me on this journey because that would include everyone I've ever met, every book I've read . . . every poem, every song, every experience. I can only try here to give thanks to those who have recently helped me with this book or been the most profound influences in my writing it.

First, I would like to thank my teachers **Robin Johnson** and **Elana Johnson**. Robin trained me in her school, Turquoise Tree Yoga Center. She is tough and kind and brilliant on many levels. She has continued to be a guiding force in my life for nearly two decades. Quite simply, she is a rock for me. I hear Elana's voice in my head. "The cream rises," she says to me when I call her with something hurting my heart, always reminding me to be graceful and extend grace to others. She is my biggest cheerleader and has never failed to be there for me.

Thank you to **Et Alia Press** for publishing *The Mud & The Lotus*, namely to my step-sister and dear friend, **Erin Wood**, for her tireless work as its editor. There are no words to express my gratitude to Erin for all she has done for me: without her there would be no book and I am forever grateful. Deep appreciation to **Amy Ashford** at Ashford Design Studio for her many hours spent thoughtfully styling the many disparate parts of this book, forging it into something unified and special. Additional appreciation to George Jensen, Kathy Oliverio, and Jacob Bozeman for their help through Et Alia.

David McBurney's captivating illustration, *Mud and the lotus*, graces this cover and captures so much of what I love about the parable, lit with my favorite color, turquoise. Thank you, David, for lending the use of your art, which spoke to Erin and me across oceans.

Elizabeth Hartzell Wood, my student and friend, is appreciated for her renderings and her patience with me as we both learned about publishing together.

I acknowledge **Meredith Finn** for her photography skills, for making me look good in pictures, and for her patience and friendship.

In attempting to thank **Rena Wren**, it is difficult to know where to start. My right hand, partner in Balance Barre, friend, student, co-teacher, a lead teacher in my school, and all around amazing person, Rena spent many months reviewing my manuscript, fact checking, making corrections, giving me her opinions and feedback about my work, and using the work to teach in the school—all while owning/running Soul Feed Yoga and serving as a traveling yoga teacher and workshop and retreat leader. Rena has traveled with me for hundreds of hours teaching in my school, assisting me and working energetically. My dear friend and confidant, she always lifts me up. I am forever grateful for this talented woman and cannot imagine making this journey without her by my side.

I thank **Larry Payne**, my Prime of Life Yoga™ Certification teacher, for his contribution to my professional life and to this book. Founding president of the International Association of Yoga Therapists (IAYT), founding director of Yoga Therapy Rx™ and Prime of Life Yoga™ programs at Loyola Marymount University, and author of many books, Larry's contribution to yoga as I know it is immense. His career is impressive by any standard and he is credited with bringing much of the world of yoga therapy to the US by his studies with leading teachers from India like Desikachar and his father, Krishnamacharya.

How lucky I am to have met **John Kepner**, Executive Director of IAYT, years ago, and to share our state of residence. I was fortunate to be invited to an international meeting of IAYT leaders at his home about 7 years prior to this book being written. For me, attending the meeting was like going to the Academy Awards. John took me under his wing and has nurtured my endeavors, mentored me, and been a steady friend. My fondest memory of our friendship was attending the IAYT Conference a few years ago, when John went out of his way to introduce me to many talented people in the world of yoga therapy. I couldn't be more grateful.

Karen Fabian and I became friends via the web. I followed her "Bare Bones Yoga" Facebook page years ago and regularly read her blog. I am ever impressed with how humble and real she is as an accomplished teacher, author of three books, and with a thriving business educating yoga teachers through webinars and online programming. Karen has assisted me with teacher trainings by offering conference calls and programs to my students. I can't thank her enough for lending her support and expertise.

With much gratitude, I would like to thank my fellow friends, students, and yoga teachers **Deby Sweatt** and **Karin Bara** for their proofing and review of my manuscript, as well as for their counsel and friendship. I trust these women implicitly. Thank you to my dear friend **Karen Gardner** who gives me a faithful listening ear, and loyally loves me.

Thank you to all the students who, during training, gave me feedback on the contents of the book. It was invaluable to witness the information being used in training and discuss how it would work in print.

Thank you **Jim**, my partner and supporter, who has undying faith in me. To my beautiful children **Will**, **Cole**, **Felisha**, and **Miller Butler** who never doubt me and always support my work. To my mother, **Frances Pennington**, who encourages me and talks me up to anyone who will listen. To my parents **Bill and Cathy High** who never fail to tell me how proud they are of me. I truly value having a loving family.

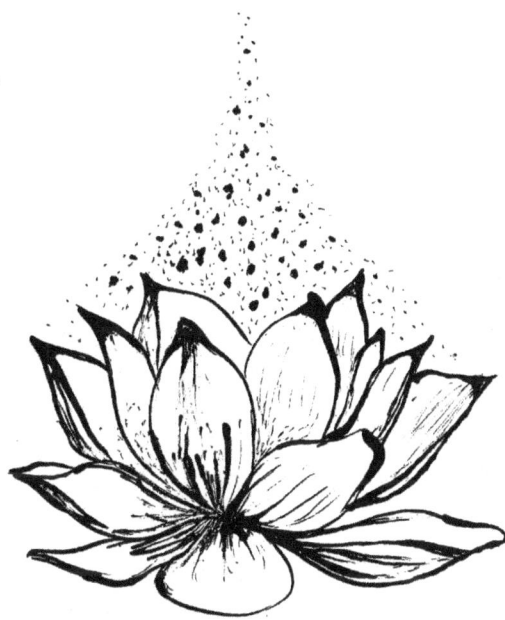

Other Titles from Et Alia Press

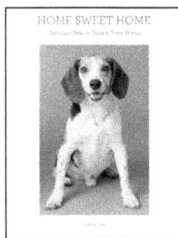

With the hope of encouraging adoption and fostering of rescue dogs, and generosity of time and treasure to local shelters and organizations, *Home Sweet Home: Arkansas Rescue Dogs & Their Stories* shares the images and stories of 26 Arkansas rescue dogs. Inspired by her own furry family members, author Grace Vest shares how a simple choice to adopt can rescue canines and humans alike.

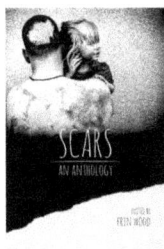

Scars: An Anthology, edited by Erin Wood, examines the range and nuance of experience related to scars of the body. Through various genres and mediums, forty contributors address self-mutilation, creating art, gender confirmation surgery, cancer, birth, brain injury, war, coming of age, pain, and love, all focusing on the central question of what it means to live with physical scars.

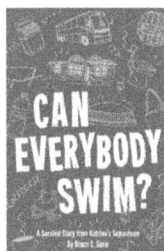

Who can forget the Louisiana Superdome? In his memoir *Can Everybody Swim? A Survival Story from Katrina's Superdome*, Bruce S. Snow takes you beyond the camera's lens on a journey through the maelstrom. A shortage of cash combined with a fierce loyalty to protect the Gentilly neighborhood family home purchased by his Ecuadorian immigrant grandparents led the then twenty-five-year-old author and his family to remain in their City to weather the storm, including enduring six days in the infamous Superdome. Follow this family of four and a half as they survive the worst natural disaster of the 21st century.

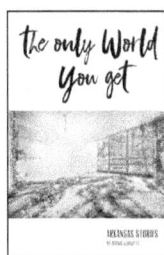

The Only World You Get collects twelve new and previously published stories, all set in Arkansas. This is the sixth collection by Dennis Vannatta, winner of Arkansas' most lucrative and prestigious literary award, The Porter Prize.

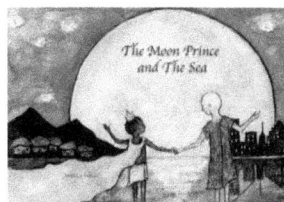

The Moon Prince and The Sea, by Dr. Daniela Rose Anderson, is based on the true story of a bond formed across an ocean between two children who found joy despite terminal illnesses. In a hospital in India, Sumit is surrounded by children who call the hospital their home; in a hospital in America, Marina is surrounded by her loving family and friends. This book is intended for children and families experiencing sickness, grief, or loss, and for any child who is curious about these topics.

For best pricing, order direct:
etaliapress.com• etaliapressbooks@gmail.com

About the Author

Courtney has been a practitioner of yoga for nearly four decades and a yoga teacher for nearly two. She delights in being of service by sharing the gift of yoga with others.

Courtney has every credential available from Yoga Alliance including the 500 E-RYT (Experienced Registered Yoga Teacher who has taught at least 1,000 hours since graduating from a Registered Yoga School), RCYT (Registered Children's Yoga Teacher), RPYT (Registered Prenatal Yoga Teacher), and YACEP (Yoga Alliance Continuing Education Provider) designations. She was one of the first yoga therapists to be recognized by the International Association of Yoga Therapists as a Certified Yoga Therapist (C-IAYT), and has been providing private yoga therapy for more than a decade. She is also trained as a Prime of Life Yoga Teacher, is a Stress Management Specialist for The Dr. Dean Ornish Reversal Program, and has earned the POLY-500 and Yoga of 12-Step Recovery (Y12SR) certifications. In her role as a certified Solution-Focused Coach (CFSC), she was a featured speaker in the 2017 Resolve to Reclaim Personal and Business Summit, and regularly offers goal-oriented coaching to clients nationwide.

A professional teacher since 2001, Courtney began leading workshops in 2006, and organizing and leading retreats in 2009. In 2008, she opened Balance Yoga and Wellness Yoga School (R.Y.S. 200/300/500 with a Yoga Alliance school rating of 4.85/5 stars) in her hometown of Hot Springs, Arkansas, and has since trained nearly 200 students through the school. She often operates Balance Yoga and Wellness Yoga School in other locations nationwide. Her experience in the yoga business also includes running her own studio, managing and creating an extensive yoga program for a 3,000+ member health and wellness nonprofit, assisting yoga studios in their planning and opening phases, and consulting studios and teachers nationwide. She has taught thousands of students and joyfully dedicated many thousands of hours to teaching. Courtney's proudest accomplishment in yoga is seeing those she has trained through Balance Yoga and Wellness go on to be successful teachers.

Courtney is mother to four grown children. She is in the midst of moving with her partner to their 40-acre Arkansas farm with many furry friends (including rescued cats, dogs, horses, and donkeys). In addition to yoga and meditation, Courtney loves being in nature (especially near water), working out, reading, and spending time with loved ones. She believes that the human condition offers us daily opportunities to revisit the parable of the mud and the lotus; as life gives us ups and downs, it always offers the practice of yoga as a lifestyle, providing us a framework for bringing ourselves back into balance and for finding happiness in the muddy waters of life.

To reach Courtney for consulting or coaching, or to learn more about Balance Yoga and Wellness Yoga School, visit her at balanceyogaandwellness.com.

"Above all Love. Love is always the answer."

Thank you for reading and engaging with *The Mud & The Lotus*.
Om, Shanti, Shanti, Shanti, Namaste.

Love and Light,
Courtney Butler

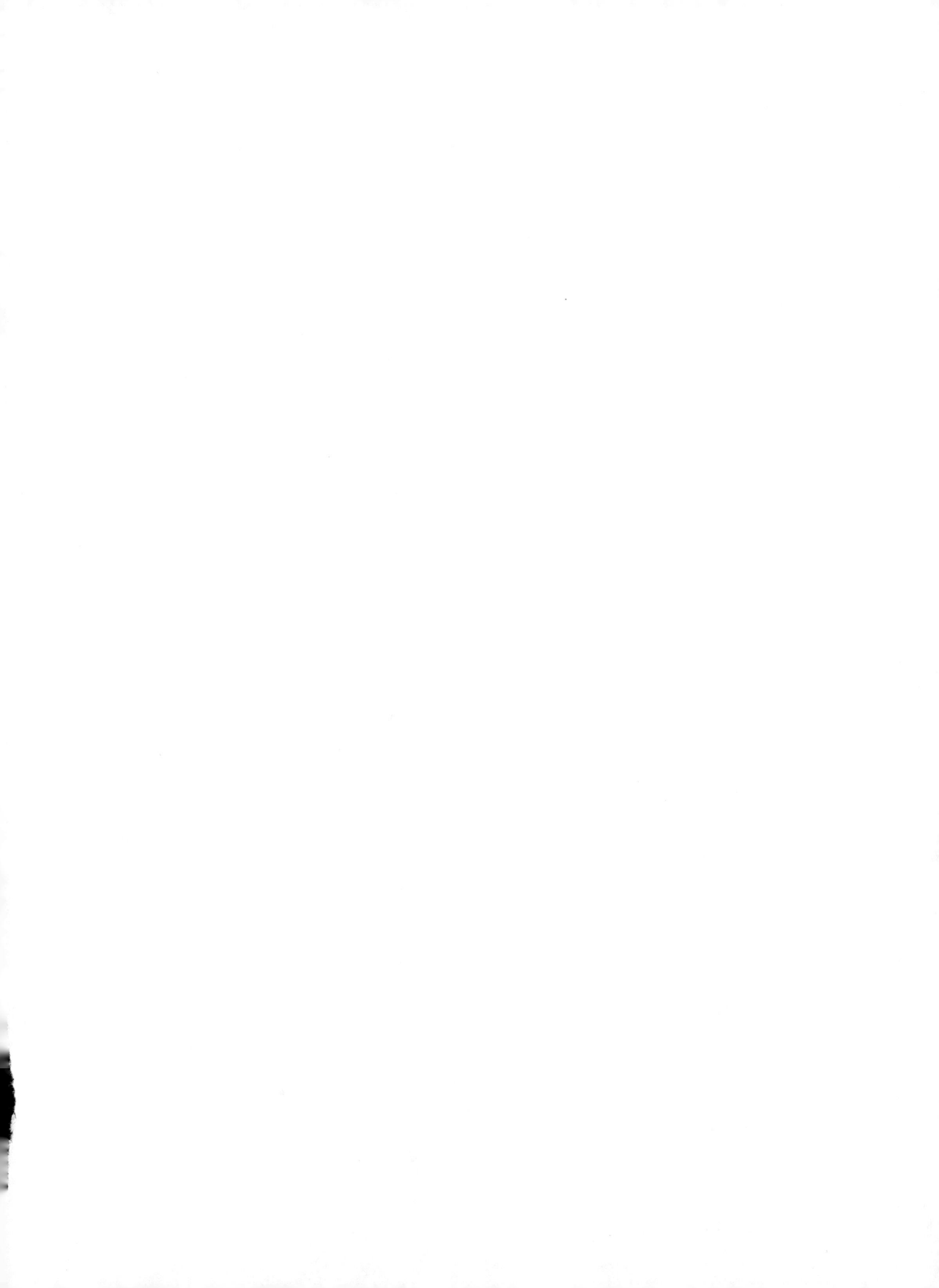

www.ingramcontent.com/pod-product-compliance
Lightning Source LLC
Chambersburg PA
CBHW080236270326
41926CB00020B/4259